GROWTH DISORDERS IN CHILDREN

GROWTH DISORDERS IN CHILDREN

J M H Buckler

Senior Lecturer and Consultant Paediatrician
The General Infirmary, Leeds

BMJ
Publishing
Group

© BMJ Publishing Group 1994

First published in 1994
by the BMJ Publishing Group, BMA House, Tavistock Square,
London WC1H 9JR

British Library Cataloguing in Publication Data

A catalogue record for this book is available
from the British Library

ISBN 0–7279–0833–2

Typeset, printed and bound in Great Britain by
Latimer Trend & Company Ltd, Plymouth

Contents

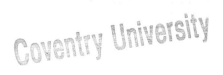

Preface

The importance of considering the growth status of a child, both as it currently is, and as it will progress through to adult life, is increasingly being emphasised within paediatrics. How a child is growing is an indication of the state of his or her health, nutrition, and wellbeing, and when growth is seen to be abnormal this observation is often the pointer that leads to the identification of a health problem and maybe to its subsequent specific diagnosis. Such an awareness of the relevance of growth impinges on the activities of many more medical personnel than just those who are experts in growth and paediatric endocrinological disorders. The need is for the non-specialist to identify children with potential growth problems early, to know how to evaluate such children at the primary care level, to know the likely short term and long term implications, physical and psychological (for the family as well as the individual), and to know what therapy is available and appropriate.

This book is designed to address these considerations at a level appropriate for such non-specialists – primarily doctors dealing with children in general practice and in the community. Usually such individuals should fulfil a role through which they can recognise the need for referral to a specialist who would be the one who would then undertake fuller investigation and determine the details of treatment when such would be considered appropriate. This manual is however also relevant to a wider range of persons involved in child care, notably health visitors and other nurses, junior hospital doctors, and paediatricians in training. It is not intended to be a fully comprehensive manual of growth and endocrinology, and for those requiring fuller information of a more specialist nature references are included. Rare disorders are not discussed in depth. Simple tables, diagrams, and illustrations are used to clarify and abbreviate the text, and the book can be used for reference as well as for continuous reading. The text refers to the British system of measurement, assessment, and treatment but much of it is universally applicable, and what is not should be interpreted in the light of the different approach in other countries.

Though many aspects of auxology may seem complex and obscure to the non-specialist, it is hoped that this book will allow the subject to be freed from the mystique sometimes attached to it, so that the simplicity of the fundamentals can be understood, accepted, and confidently applied by all those for whom the subject is relevant. A non-expert practitioner need not be inhibited by ignorance of the esoteric aspects and minutiae of this subject of growth.

1: Normal growth

What is normality?

The majority of children would be considered by most people – medical and otherwise – to be growing normally, and only a minority would be considered to be unequivocally abnormal in their growth. However, there are a significant number about whom opinions will vary, depending on differing criteria, standards, and knowledge. These judgments will be influenced by such aspects as family expectancy and pattern of growth, general health and wellbeing, and whether psychological, emotional, or social difficulties arise as a result of the growth status. It is impossible to define "normal" growth, for the variation within a population is vast, in terms of the range of size of the measurements, their interrelationships, and the timing of growth episodes (notably puberty). These aspects are considered in Chapters 3–5, and in Chapter 7 those pointers are discussed that would give rise to concern about a growth pattern or suggest that it might be abnormal.

Average growth

It is clear that "average" and "normal" are far from synonymous, but nevertheless it is of value to be aware of the average growth pattern of a boy or girl, for there are misconceptions as to what may be expected even with this. Figure 4.2 (p. 40) shows these expected changes in weight and length or height through childhood, Table 7.2 (p. 72) those specific to the early years of life.

Centile charts

The first essential requirement for interpreting growth is to have standards that form a basis for comparison. These standards are depicted on growth centile charts, which show the spread of measurements within a large, assumedly normal, population through an age range of the growing period of life. Figures are assigned to each line, indicating the percentage of boys or girls whose values would fall below that particular line in a comparable population. Most commonly the 3rd, 10th, 25th,

50th, 75th, 90th, and 97th centiles are shown. There is no particular centile representing the divide between normality and abnormality, for many other factors must be taken into consideration (see Chapter 7), but, in general, the further a measurement is from the average at a given age, the more likely there is to be a problem, and the identification of a child's centile is the first step in the evaluation of his or her growth, and leads on to other considerations. For measurements based on bony structures, such as height, there is a symmetrical (Gaussian) distribution around the mean within the normal population, and for such measurements it is often convenient to think in terms of standard deviations. The relationship between centiles and standard deviation for values with

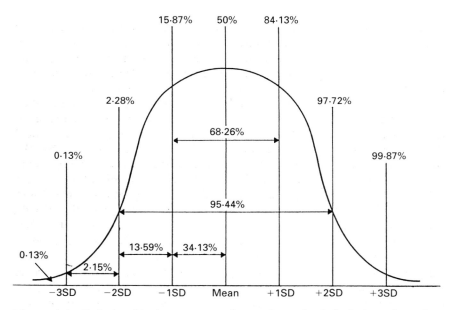

Figure 1.1 Relationship between centiles and standard deviations for values with a Gaussian distribution

a symmetrical distribution is shown in Figure 1.1 and Table 1.1. Centiles for measurements, such as weight and skinfolds, that do not show an even distribution cannot so readily be expressed as standard deviations.

Centile charts are derived from a particular population at a particular period in time and, strictly speaking, may not be ideal for the interpretation of growth of other individuals, or groups of a different race

Table 1.1 Approximate relationships for height between standard deviations and centiles

Standard deviation	Centile	Proportion taller or shorter within the population
+3	99·9	1 in 750 taller
+2·5	99	1 in 100 taller
+2	97	1 in 44 taller
+1	84	1 in 6 taller
0	50	Equal numbers taller or shorter
−1	16	1 in 6 shorter
−2	3	1 in 44 shorter
−2·5	1	1 in 100 shorter
−3	0·1	1 in 750 shorter

or geographical location, or in later years. The pattern of growth of a population of any age does change over time; children (and adults) have tended to get taller and heavier through the course of this century, and, ideally, updated standards should be produced regularly. This, however, is a major undertaking and the first new set of centile charts for over 20 years has only recently been produced.[1] It is of interest that, when comparing the new centiles with the old, differences are not as great as might have been anticipated, neither in the overall trend, nor in regional differences within the United Kingdom. The inference here is that the secular trend, so apparent earlier in the century, is now slowing down. The latest standards show a difference in height of only about 1·5 cm between the extremes regionally, the children being tallest in the South of England and becoming progressively smaller towards the North, though Welsh children are the shortest of all. The values for the 3rd, 50th, and 97th centiles of the Tanner standards[2] dated 1975, superimposed on the new ones for boys' and girls' weights and heights are shown in Figure 1.2a–d. The differences appear most obvious over the years covering puberty; however, caution should be used in interpreting the new charts since they are cross sectional and do not yet include longitudinal data and are therefore of restricted applicability to that age range. Little change is evident over the period of infant growth.[3] The overall change from the last Tanner standards dated 1975[2] is an increase of only about 1·5 cm in mid-childhood, and less for adults. These previous values were, however, based on children in Southern England and slightly overestimated the stature for the country as a whole, yet they remain a satisfactory basic standard. The newest standards are based on samples from the whole of the British mainland.[1] Although it is not practical to have separate standards for different ethnic groups or geographical areas

3

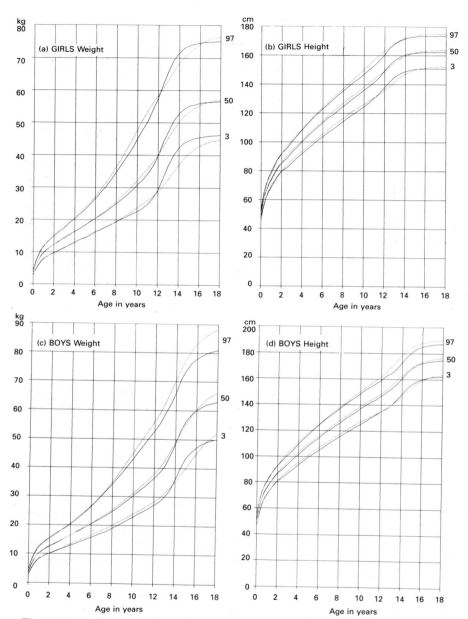

Figure 1.2   Comparison of old and new data. (a) Girls' weight; (b) girls' height; (c) boys' weight; (d) boys' height. (———) Data from 1975[2]; (⋯⋯⋯⋯) data from 1994[1]

within a country, it is important at an initial observation to be aware that these factors may be relevant in interpreting centile positions.

Centile charts thus not only form the basis for assessing the growth of an *individual*, but also compare the distribution of measurements of groups from different geographical areas or from different ethnic, cultural, or socioeconomic backgrounds. Centile charts show the status of the population from which they were derived as they actually were at the time, not necessarily as they ideally should have been. In practice the charts in common use in this country are considered to be derived from a "normal", and by general assumption "ideal", population. However, when the "standard" population does not have optimal status, for instance where there is large scale malnutrition, the distribution represented may be far from ideal.

Centile charts have also been produced from populations of individuals with specific pathologies sufficiently common to justify the undertaking, notably Down's syndrome and Turner's syndrome, and these enable interpretation of the growth of an individual within the overall spectrum of that condition as well as using standard "normal" charts for reference.

The sources of the centile charts in use at the present time are listed in Appendix 2.

Distance centiles

These show how actual measurements, such as height, weight, head circumference, etc, progress with age, and show at any particular age the cumulative outcome of all the previous growth.

Velocity centiles

Velocity centiles show the rate of change – the amount a measurement increases (or occasionally, as with weight, decreases) over the course of time, usually per year. These standards show the range of growth rates found within a large, normal population. Contrary to what might be expected, however, the spread of "normal" velocities over a prolonged period of time is not such that 3% of the normal population would have velocities below the 3rd centile nor 3% above the 97th centile. By definition they will show this range for short periods as growth velocities vary considerably short term in normal children. The way in which velocities, long term, correspond to the "distance" centiles is shown in

5

Table 1.2 *Equivalence between height centiles and height velocity centiles*

Height centile	Height velocity centile
3	25
50	50
97	75

Table 1.3 *Merits of estimating velocities on the basis of observations over different periods*

	Over a full year	Shorter term, for example 3–6 monthly
Effect of errors in measurement and other variations (for example, time of day)	Minimal	Exaggerated
Frequency of obtainable values	Initial need to wait a year, but subsequently as frequent as clinic visits	At every clinic visit
Effect of seasonal variations	Obliterated	Evident
Recognition of short term changes, for example due to: progression of illness, response to treatment, or stages of rapid growth, (infancy, puberty)	Obscured	Evident

Table 1.2. Velocities remaining outside the 25th–75th centile range for a prolonged period will indicate growth deviating from the centiles and will thus be a pointer that there may be some underlying problem, except at puberty (see Chapter 6). Minor deviations from a height centile line are not always easy to see by eye over intervals as short as a year or so, and slow or fast growth will therefore be identified more clearly on a height velocity chart. *As a rule of thumb, before the age at which the consideration of puberty becomes relevant (see Chapter 6) children growing "normally" have heights and weights that basically adhere to a centile line and therefore have velocities that lie between the 25th and 75th centiles.*

Estimation of velocities

Velocities are recorded as a change in a measurement over a period of a year. This may indeed represent the increase from a time in one

Table 1.4   Calendar of decimal dates

	1 Jan.	2 Feb.	3 Mar.	4 Apr.	5 May	6 June	7 July	8 Aug.	9 Sept.	10 Oct.	11 Nov.	12 Dec.
1	000	085	162	247	329	414	496	581	666	748	833	915
2	003	088	164	249	332	416	499	584	668	751	836	918
3	005	090	167	252	334	419	501	586	671	753	838	921
4	008	093	170	255	337	422	504	589	674	756	841	923
5	011	096	173	258	340	425	507	592	677	759	844	926
6	014	C99	175	260	342	427	510	595	679	762	847	929
7	016	101	178	263	345	430	512	597	682	764	849	932
8	019	104	181	266	348	433	515	600	685	767	852	934
9	022	107	184	268	351	436	518	603	688	770	855	937
10	025	110	186	271	353	438	521	605	690	773	858	940
11	027	112	189	274	356	441	523	608	693	775	860	942
12	030	115	192	277	359	444	526	611	696	778	863	945
13	033	118	195	279	362	447	529	614	699	781	866	948
14	036	121	197	282	364	449	532	616	701	784	868	951
15	038	123	200	285	367	452	534	619	704	786	871	953
16	041	126	203	288	370	455	537	622	707	789	874	956
17	044	129	205	290	373	458	540	625	710	792	877	959
18	047	132	208	293	375	460	542	627	712	795	879	962
19	049	134	211	296	378	463	545	630	715	797	882	964
20	052	137	214	299	381	466	548	633	718	800	885	967
21	055	140	216	301	384	468	551	636	721	803	888	970
22	058	142	219	304	386	471	553	638	723	805	890	973
23	060	145	222	307	389	474	556	641	726	808	893	975
24	063	148	225	310	392	477	559	644	729	811	896	978
25	066	151	227	312	395	479	562	647	731	814	899	981
26	068	153	230	315	397	482	564	649	734	816	901	984
27	071	156	233	318	400	485	567	652	737	819	904	986
28	074	159	236	321	403	488	570	655	740	822	907	989
29	077		238	323	405	490	573	658	742	825	910	992
30	079		241	326	408	493	575	660	745	827	912	995
31	082		244		411		578	663		830		997

year to the same time the next year, or can be estimated on the basis of observations at shorter intervals multiplied up by the appropriate factor, as if that rate of growth had persisted for a full year.

There are advantages and disadvantages to these two methods of estimating velocities, as indicated in Table 1.3. In order to make these calculations, ages and intervals must be worked out on the basis of "decimals". Table 1.4 shows the calendar of dates as decimals or the number of thousandths all the way through the year.

A decimal age is the date in decimals at the time of observation minus the birth date in decimals.

Table 1.5 Example of a child's height velocity

Date of observation	Decimal date	Decimal age (years)	Height (cm)	Height increment (cm)		Time interval (year)		Height velocity (cm/year)	
				Over 4 months	Over 1 year	4 months	1 year	Over 4 months	Over 1 year
5 December 1986	86·926	Birth							
4 October 1992	92·756	92·756 − 86·926 = 5·83	101·5						
23 January 1993	93·060	93·060 − 86·926 = 6·13	102·3	102·3 − 101·5 = 0·8		6·13 − 5·83 = 0·30		0·8/0·3 = 2·7	
15 May 1993	93·367	93·367 − 86·926 = 6·44	104·2	104·2 − 102·3 = 1·9		6·44 − 6·13 = 0·31		1·9/0·31 = 6·1	
10 October 1993	93·773	93·773 − 86·926 = 6·85	106·4	106·4 − 104·2 = 2·1	106·4 − 101·5 = 4·9	6·85 − 6·44 = 0·41	6·85 − 5·83 = 1·02	2·2/0·41 = 5·4	4·9/ 1·02 = 4·8

The decimal interval between measurements is the age in decimals at time (1) minus the age in decimals at time (2).

The velocity (for example cm/year) is given by:

$$\frac{\text{Measurement at time (1) minus measurement at time (2)}}{\text{Decimal interval between time (1) and time (2).}}$$

Table 1.5 illustrates this method.

Cross sectional and longitudinal data

Centile charts can be compiled by observations on one occasion only of many individuals over the desired age range, giving cross sectional data. They may also be based on repetitive measurements on the same individuals (inevitably smaller numbers) over prolonged periods of time, giving longitudinal data. In the age range between infancy and puberty, when velocities are relatively steady, there is little difference in the picture produced by these two methods. However, at times of rapidly changing velocities (such as puberty) the two methods will produce very differently shaped curves because the age of the changes within the normal population is so variable. This is illustrated in Figure 1.3. The pooled cross sectional data are quite unlike the actual growth rate of any individual. Centile charts covering these periods usually include curves representing the actual shape for individuals, and the composite to indicate the spread of the age range at which these changes may happen.[4]

For any individual the shape of the velocity curve through the years will vary greatly, depending on whether the observations are based on short intervals, for example 4 months, or intervals of a full year. Figure 1.4 shows an example of this.

Sex differences

There is little difference in the centiles of height and weight of boys and girls, and the corresponding velocities, prior to the onset of puberty. At puberty, however, because the timing of growth changes is so different between the sexes, the measurements differ markedly and progressively as illustrated in Figure 1.5[5] and considered more fully in Chapter 6.

9

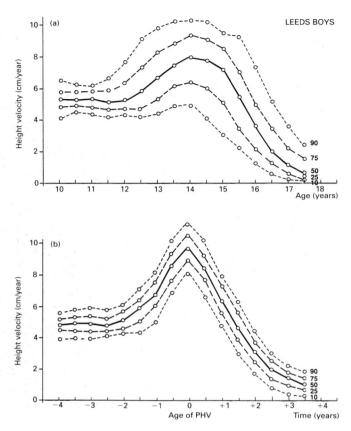

Figure 1.3   Height velocity charts showing (a) cross sectional and (b) lon-gitudinal data[5]

Different concepts of age

The terminology "age" for various parameters in addition to "actual" age is sometimes used in describing growth status; some of these para-meters are listed in Box A. These concepts are sometimes of value in comparing how the degree of deviation from the average varies in relation to different parameters of growth, but they can be misleading as these characteristics do not necessarily change in parallel, particularly at the time of puberty.

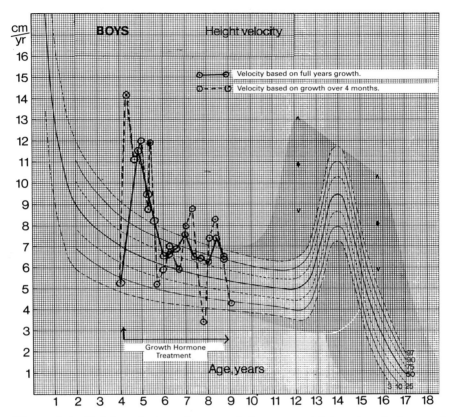

Figure 1.4 Height velocity of a growth hormone deficient boy before and during treatment

11

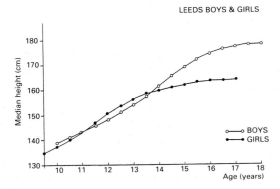

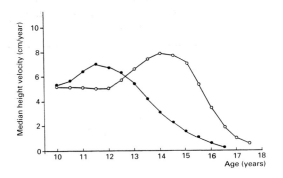

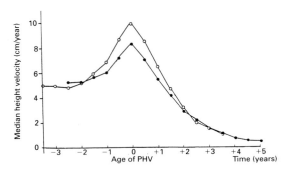

Figure 1.5 Height and height velocity graphs to compare the growth of boys and girls at around the time of puberty[5]

Box A: Some definitions of age

Chronological age
(= calendar age)

Actual age as the time between observation date and date of birth.

Height or weight age

Age at which the individual's height or weight would correspond with the 50th centile on the standard charts for the population of that sex.

Skeletal (bone) age
(see Chapter 5)

Average age within the normal population to which the bony development of the individual corresponds.

Pubertal age

Average age within the normal population (50th centile) of that sex to which the pubertal status of the individual corresponds.

2: Assessment of growth

There is a surprising lack of agreement among paediatricians and growth experts about many aspects of growth assessment, including the value, timing, and method of routine growth surveillance, the most appropriate methods of measurement and equipment, the criteria indicating the need for further action, and what that action should be and by whom it should be taken.

Table 2.1 Stages of growth assessment

Stage	Indication	Method
1 Initial measurement	Routine screening On basis of concern	Appropriate techniques for appropriate parameters
2 Recording		Correct documentation in available form and accurate plotting on centile charts
3 Interpretation		See text (Chapters 1 and 7)
4 Action	If no concern If possible concern If great concern	Continuing routine check Specific planned follow up to aid evaluation Referral for fuller assessment

The stages of growth assessment are indicated in Table 2.1. These are basically obvious, but nevertheless neglect or error can happen at any stage, resulting either in a child with a real growth problem being missed or overinvolvement with one in whom concern is inappropriate.

Routine screening measurements

The value of routine measurements at regular intervals is that children with growth problems can be identified at an early stage while there is sufficient time available for effective outcome from treatment for those who need it. Unfortunately many children are not identified as abnormally short or tall until they are close to puberty or it is under way, whereas recognition of the problem in earlier childhood, when frequently it was already evident, would have allowed time for the child to benefit from much longer treatment. Ideally the poor growth associated with congenital conditions should be identified within the first 5 years, which is seldom the case at present. However, as Table 2.1 indicates, it is not sufficient merely to undertake the measurements and to record and plot them on centile charts, but it is necessary to take appropriate action. Even in those children in whom routine measurements do not suggest a problem at the time, such observations are worthwhile in that they provide a baseline for comparison with subsequent measurements when the child is older and growth may be giving cause for concern. *Reliable measurements on record are invaluable for later comparison.*

Timing of routine measurements

The Hall Report[6] recommends routine height measurement at around 3 years of age (or earlier if the child is cooperative) and between 4 and 5 years, only advocating further measurements if these give cause for concern. The report considers that there is no justification for routine weighing of children beyond the first year of life. In my opinion there is a place for more frequent routine measurements of both weight and height or length, for the value of the information from either alone is increased by a comparison of the two. Clearly, in making re-commendations, one may have to compromise between what is optimal and what is realistic, and this perforce will vary depending on the availability of staff, their training and ability, and the type of population and its willingness to comply. There are several reasons why meas-urements may be unreliable, as indicated in Box A. As long as potential

---

Box A: Reasons for unreliability of measurements
Inaccuracy
- Faulty technique – inexperienced, untrained staff
- Faulty equipment – wrongly positioned or calibrated
- Uncooperative children.

Different observers
Different times of day

---

errors are not too great, these effects will not matter much with regard to conclusions drawn from initial observations, but they do become crucial when comparing sequential observations, although the longer the interval between measurements, the less is the significance of errors. However, over short periods such as 3 months or less (between the ages of 2 and puberty) the magnitude of these "errors" may actually approximate to the correct change in height over that period. Incorrect observations will therefore result in incorrect conclusions that would invalidate any theoretical benefit from frequent visits.

Table 2.2   Proposed programme of routine measuring

Age	Height/length	Weight	Head circumference
6 weeks	*	√	√
3 months	*	√	√
6–9 months	*	√	√
12–15 months	*	√	√
2 years	√	√	√
3 years	√	√	
4–5 years	√	√	
7 years	√	√	
9 years	√	√	
11 years	√	√	
13 years	√	√	

* Length should be measured at these visits if reliable facilities are available and particularly if there is any doubt regarding the adequacy of weight gain

A realistic timetable for routine measurements is suggested in Table 2.2. Many of these times are selected to coincide with those of routine health checks or immunisation, but clearly opportunistic use of contact with children to measure them when they are seen at other times for other reasons should not be missed. The information should, however, be collated in a readily available health record if the best use is to be made of the observations, for example parent-held records or general practitioner records. It may later be invaluable to have such reliable measurements on record.

It is clearly of importance to determine who should have the overall responsibility for these growth measurements and, as part of the overall Child Health Surveillance programme, general practitioners will frequently be the best placed. However, excellent community growth screening projects are being undertaken in many places by health visitors and school nurses under the supervision of community paediatricians, and hopefully, in time, they will be in a position to check that the programmes are implemented.

Check ups based on initial anxiety

Deviations of growth may not only be identified as a result of routine surveillance, but also at the instigation of individuals who for various reasons feel anxious about a child's growth. The possible sources of such concern are listed in Box B, and the reasons why they are concerned in Box C. However, parental anxiety about children's growth is often unnecessary and explanation of the centile positions will help to resolve many queries. *Good growth is an excellent overall indicator of general wellbeing.*

Box B: Who are the people concerned about the child's growth?

- The child?
- The parents?
- Friends and relations?
- The school staff?
- Doctors and nurses?
- Society and the media?

Box C: Why are they concerned?

- Because there is a fear that there is something fundamentally wrong.
  (Is there an underlying pathology?)
- Because of the adverse effects on the child *now*.
  (Psychological, social, emotional, physical)
- Because of fear of long-term consequences.
  (What will be the size and shape and function when fully grown?)

Measuring equipment

All equipment should be checked regularly for zero settings and for accuracy using a standard length metal rod (usually 50 cm) for height and length equipment.

Height

The best equipment for measuring height is the Harpenden Stadiometer, but this is too expensive and substantial for routine use outside a hospital setting. Many cheaper portable stadiometer devices are available (see Appendix 1), of which the Minimetre and the Leicester Height Measure are probably the most acceptable. It is important that all these devices are set up at the correct level, and on a non-carpeted floor. There is little value in height measurements undertaken by placing a book on the head, or using cheap measuring sticks. Wall mounted screening charts (see Appendix 1) are available which serve as a guide for levels of concern and referral, but they provide no permanent record and their use alone is not recommended. These show the levels of two standard deviations, outside which referral may be considered, and three standard deviations, when referral is definitely indicated.

Length

Accurate measurements require substantial and expensive equipment, but cheaper portable forms (see Appendix 1) are adequate if used optimally and interpreted cautiously, accepting the limits of accuracy. Measurements with a tape measure alone are so inaccurate as to be useless.

Weight

The best portable scales are electronic forms (see Appendix 1) but these are heavy and expensive, and high quality bathroom scales (frequently checked) may be adequate (recognising that extreme accuracy of body weight has limited value owing to the considerable normal variation from hour to hour and day to day). Many centres may find it justifiable to purchase substantial balance scales.

Tape measures

Flexible, narrow, metal tape measures are the most reliable, but are not always as easy to apply as the fabric alternatives when measuring the head circumferences of wriggly infants. Fabric measures may stretch with time, but are not expensive to replace.

Measuring techniques

These are fully described by Cameron.[7]

Height

The subject should stand, without shoes, legs together, as tall and straight as possible, on a non-carpeted floor, ensuring that the heels stay firmly on the ground and the back and heels are in contact with the measuring device. Head tilt is avoided by ensuring that the child looks straight ahead so that the external angle of the eye is at the same level as the external auditory meatus (Frankfurt plane). The child is then stretched gently by upward pressure over the mastoids, and instructed to relax the shoulders. The sliding headpiece is lowered to rest firmly on the head and measurements should be recorded to the nearest millimetre. Certain types of hairstyle may present difficulties!

Length

Measurements cannot be achieved without two people, one to hold the head against the fixed head piece, and the other stretching the legs of the supine infant, ensuring that they and the body are straight, and holding the feet at right angles to the legs. The best devices have a sliding footpiece which is brought into firm contact with the heels and soles and the length is recorded to the nearest millimetre.

Weight

Babies should be weighed unclothed, and toddlers and older children in only light underclothes, to the nearest 0·1 kg. Care should be taken to ensure that they do not touch any objects alongside the scales.

Head circumference

Measurements should be taken around the maximum occipitofrontal diameter to the nearest millimetre.

Mid-upper arm circumference

Measurements are taken at the midpoint of the left upper arm with the arm hanging by the side. The tape should not compress the tissues.

Skinfold measurements

These measurements show the thickness of subcutaneous tissue and primarily reflect fat. Although they will probably not be routinely under- taken, they are simple to carry out using reliable skinfold calipers. Most calipers measure to 0·1 mm over a range of 0–48 mm. Skinfolds can be measured at several sites, but the two most commonly used (for which centile charts are available), which probably reflect best the body fat component as a whole, are the triceps and subscapular. The triceps skinfold is measured at the midpoint of the mid-posterior line of the left upper arm with the arm extended and hanging loosely at the side. The subscapular skinfold is measured vertically, directly below the angle of the left scapula.

The caliper is held with the right hand, and a fold of skin and subcutaneous tissue is lifted up from the underlying muscle between the thumb and index finger of the left hand. The jaws of the caliper are applied directly below to enclose this skinfold and the distance between is read directly from the dial within a few seconds.

Body proportions

The relationship of the length of the trunk to that of the limbs is occasionally a pointer to underlying pathology (see Chapter 7). It is seldom practical outside a hospital setting to obtain accurate values for these components but as a rough guide, which may identify extremes of disproportion, the following simple techniques can be used.

Sitting height

The subject sits on a hard, flat, horizontal surface, such as a narrow table, so that the back is against a wall and in contact with it, in a similar way to that for the measurement of height. Ideally, the legs should be positioned so that the backs of the knees are in contact with the edge of the table over which the legs hang loosely (in practice, the width of the table will seldom be such as to make this possible, unless a very expensive sitting height table is used). The subject sits as tall as possible, without shrugging the shoulders, and traction is applied upwards on the mastoids as for measurement of height. A second person identifies the level of the top of the head using, for example, a stiff book horizontally placed, and the height from the top of the table to this level is measured with a tape measure. It is to be stressed that such a technique is very approximate, only to be used on a one-off basis and not accurate enough for serial observations, and a similar method without appropriate equipment should never be used for measuring height.

Subischial leg length

This is calculated as height minus sitting height. Centile charts are available for sitting height and leg length.

Span

This is the measurement from fingertip to fingertip. The subject stands erect with back against the wall, arms outstretched horizontally and palms of hands facing forwards. One observer holds the fingertips of one hand against a wall corner, while gently stretching the arms. (The degree to which the arms are stretched cannot be precisely controlled, hence the approximate nature of this measurement.) An assistant marks on the wall the position of the middle fingertip of the other hand. The distance between the wall corner and this mark is then measured with a tape measure to the nearest half centimetre, as greater accuracy is unrealistic.

The ratios of these measurements clearly vary greatly within the normal population and with age, but approximate means are shown in Table 2.3. Infants have proportionately short limbs and large head and trunks and these proportions gradually change through childhood to adult values (with the "hiccup" at puberty) as indicated in the table. The proportions change dramatically through the course of puberty as shown in Figure 2.1. (Owing to the great range of age at which puberty can occur, the ages in this figure are based on a common pubertal status – age of peak height velocity (PHV) – rather than actual age.)

21

In individuals on whom it is technically difficult to perform measurements of full stature, for example, those with paraplegia, severe arthritis, or spinal deformities, the measurement of span or sitting height may be an alternative means to indicate what the "stature ought to be."

Table 2.3   Approximate mean ratios of sitting height and limb lengths

Ratio	Both sexes			Male			Female		
Age in years	Birth	2	5	10	Age of PHV	Adult	10	Age of PHV	Adult
Sitting height/height	0·60	0·57	0·55	0·535	0·517	0·528	0·535	0·527	0·534
Sitting height/leg length	1·54	1·31	1·21	1·15	1·07	1·12	1·155	1·11	1·15
Span/height		0·992	0·995	0·996	0·998	1·010	1·017	0·993	1·001	1·006

PHV = Peak height velocity

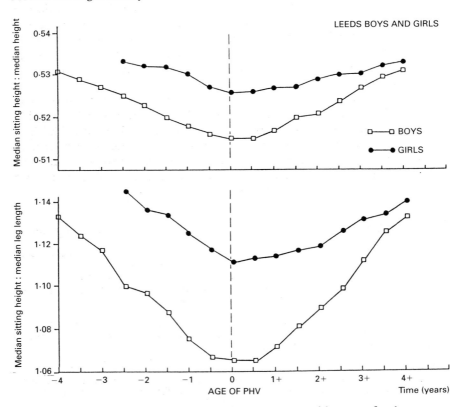

Figure 2.1   Ratios of body proportions at comparable ages of puberty

Pubertal status

Chapter 6 stresses the extreme importance of noting the stage of sexual development at all ages when it might be relevant, for this is essential for the correct interpretation of growth patterns. The stages of puberty as described by Tanner,[8,9] and used almost universally, are shown in Figures 2.2 and 2.3.

Recommended action on the basis of growth observations

The clinical pointers to abnormal growth are outlined in Chapter 7, but preliminary guidelines are indicated in Table 2.4. Interpretation of the height centile position alone may be misleading, as the expected position is dependent on the height of the parents, and the correct acceptable range of height is within two standard deviations of the mid-parental centile line rather than the standard centiles (see Chapter 3, Box D (p. 32)).

Children with problems of poor growth but who have tall parents may have heights that lie well above the third centile, and it will probably take several years for fall off to bring the height below that level. Children with short parents will not be expected to be tall, and their "normal" heights will clearly be at a lower centile range than the average population. However, the possibility of an inherited cause of abnormal growth must not be forgotten when using this guideline.

Table 2.4   *Basis for referral for children (aged 2–10 years) suspected of having a growth problem*

Measurement	Indication for referral
1 Plot height centile at initial observation	Height deviates by more than three standard deviations
2 Plot range of expected height as ± 10 cm from mid-parental centile (which is equivalent to 3rd and 97th centile for this child)	Height deviates by more than two standard deviations corrected for parents' heights
3 Remeasure after 6 months and 1 year to find height velocity (over 1 year) and plot on velocity centile	Height deviates by more than two standard deviations for age together with low/high velocity

Girls: breast development

Stage 1 Preadolescent: elevation of the papilla only.

Stage 2 Breast bud stage. Elevation of the breast and papilla as a small mound. Enlargement of the areola diameter.

Stage 3 Further enlargement and elevation of the breast and areola, with no separation of their contours.

Stage 4 Projection of the areola and papilla above the level of the breast.

Stage 5 Mature stage, projection of the papilla alone due to recession of the areola.

Girls: pubic hair

Stage 1 Preadolescent: no pubic hair.

Stage 2 Sparse growth of slightly pigmented downy hair chiefly along the labia.

Stage 3 Hair darker, coarser and more curled, spreading sparsely over the junction of the pubes.

Stage 4 Hair adult in type, but covering a considerably smaller area than in the adult. No spread to the medial surface of the thighs.

Stage 5 Adult quantity and type with distribution of a horizontal pattern and spread to the medial surface of the thighs. Spread up the linea alba sometimes occurs but is late and rated Stage 6.

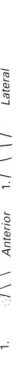
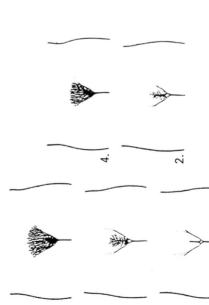

Figure 2.2   Pubertal stages: girls

24

Boys: genital development

Stage 1 Preadolescent: the testes, scrotum and penis are about the same size and proportions as in early childhood.

Stage 2 Enlargement of the scrotum and testes. The skin of the scrotum reddens and changes in texture. Little or no enlargement of the penis.

Stage 3 Lengthening of the penis. Further growth of the testes and scrotum.

Stage 4 Increase in breadth of the penis and development of the glans. The testes and scrotum are larger; the scrotum darkens.

Stage 5 Adult.

Boys: pubic hair

Stage 1 Preadolescent: no pubic hair.

Stage 2 Sparse growth of slightly pigmented downy hair chiefly at the base of the penis.

Stage 3 Hair darker, coarser and more curled, spreading over the junction of the pubes.

Stage 4 Hair adult in type, but covering a considerably smaller area than in the adult. No spread to the medial surface of the thighs.

Stage 5 Adult quantity and type with distribution of a horizontal pattern and spread to the medial surface of the thighs. Spread up the linea alba is late and rated Stage 6.

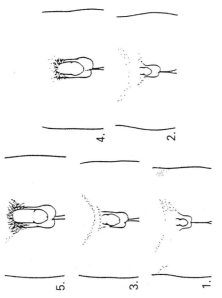

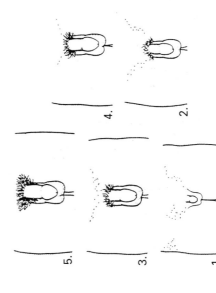

Figure 2.3   Pubertal stages: boys

25

Infants under 2 years of age

This topic is discussed in Chapter 7 (pp. 71–75). The basic criterion of evaluation of growth in infants is weight. Unfortunately, as supine length is difficult to measure because babies and infants are particularly "stretchy" and the measurement requires two people, this observation is commonly omitted, and rightly so if accuracy is likely to be very poor and the values obtained therefore misleading. However, with experience and training, length measurements need not be so inaccurate, and this extra information is of great value, as indicated in Chapter 3, in identifying the very short infant, and in aiding diagnosis of short children when assessed at a later age.

Follow up of borderline subjects

Serial measurements

Those children whose growth is not sufficiently abnormal to fulfil the first two criteria of Table 2.4, but nevertheless remain of concern, should be followed up with more regular and frequent measurements, perhaps every six months. For these serial measurements to be as comparable as possible, they should preferably be undertaken by the same observer (because there is commonly a degree of interobserver difference between experienced, competent measurers) and at approximately the same time of day. This will allow a height velocity to be calculated over a period of a year, thus lessening any effect from inaccurate measurements (see Table 1.3 (p. 6)). These sequential measurements should be continued for longer if doubt remains. Table 1.2 (p. 6) indicates the normal velocity centiles expected over a period of a year or more, according to the height centile, and so indicates the velocities which would result in deviations from the height centile position for that child, justifying referral.

If velocities are correctly interpreted, their use overcomes the problems of allowing for parental size, and racial and geographical differences in growth. However, velocity charts are only helpful between the ages of 2 and 10 years, when normal velocities are relatively steady. Between birth and 2 years of age, when velocities are normally falling very rapidly, the weight and length of normal babies frequently cross centiles before settling at their appropriate "genetic" level (see p. 29). After the age of 10 the variation in the timing of the normal pubertal growth spurt makes identification of abnormal velocities very difficult.

Weight–height correlation and interpretation

Another aspect of evaluation which may be helpful is the degree of fatness or thinness, or weight–height relationship, which is discussed in Chapter 4. In infants and young children the descriptive term "failure to thrive", discussed in Chapter 7, is frequently used, and in support of this "diagnosis" the measurement of mid-upper arm circumference may be of value (Table 2.5).

Table 2.5   Measurement of mid-upper arm circumference

Age (months)	Mid-upper arm circumference (cm)	
12–60	14–15	Warrants some concern.
	< 14	Warrants serious concern.
60	15–16	Warrants some concern.
	< 15	Warrants serious concern.

Occipitofrontal head circumference

This measurement, in infancy, provides information about overall growth of bony structures, in addition to reflecting growth of the brain. It should initially be measured soon after birth (though not immediately due to scalp oedema and moulding). This provides a useful baseline and is of value if there are developmental problems. The centile should be compared with those of length and weight, but noting that the commonest cause of large or small heads is not pathological but familial, and the measurement seldom matters if development and behaviour are normal. If in doubt, the measurement should be followed serially to find whether it is adhering to or deviating from its centile position. In usual circumstances, head circumference measurements are seldom worthwhile after the age of 2, as head growth is subsequently very slow.

3: Influences on growth

The height and weight of an individual, during the growing years and ultimately, are dependent on many interacting factors. The differences in size of members of populations comparable in age and sex are usually dependent on factors which by most people's standards would not be

---

Box A: Factors which influence in a normal way the growth status of a child

Feature	Clinical clue
"Normal" inheritance	Size of parents
"Physiological age"	Pubertal status (and bone
(see Chapter 5)	age) in relation to actual age
"Normal" variations in	Height/weight relationships;
nutritional state	skinfolds

---

considered abnormal, the more obvious of which are shown in Box A. Thus, most individuals within a population will be normal with regard to their growth, however tall or short, or fat or thin they may be (see Chapter 1, p. 1 for what is meant by "normal"). It is only in a minority of individuals that a pathological state accounts for a growth pattern which deviates from this normal range, but it is clearly of the utmost importance to recognise the clues that would suggest who these are (see Chapter 7). Box B lists conditions and circumstances which can affect growth adversely. Most of these are, or are related to growth promoting factors, but in normally growing individuals they are appropriate in their nature or quantity and only produce problems when they deviate from this norm.

Relevant clinical observations in relation to growth disorders

Size at birth and antenatal factors

Antenatal growth, like postnatal growth, is influenced by many of the factors just described, so variation in the size at birth of babies of common sex and gestational age may or may not be normal. Centile charts are available for length, weight, and head circumference at birth,

Box B: Factors which may cause short stature in pathological situations

Feature	Clinical clue
Adverse antenatal influences	Size at birth in relation to gestational age
Inherited pathological conditions	Family history
Undernutrition (inadequate intake or absorption)	Low weight for height; skinfolds
Chronic ill health	History and examination
Hormonal imbalance	Clinical picture – notably low height for weight
Adverse psychosocial conditions	History; inappropriate behaviour
"Syndromes" of short stature	Odd appearance; abnormal body proportions

plotted against gestational age, and these provide the means to judge the "appropriateness" of a newborn baby's measurements. The spread is similar to that expected in interpreting postnatal growth centile charts. The height of the mother will influence the length of a newborn baby. Subsequently the part played by the father's height becomes evident also, so that by the age of 2 the height of the child should have adjusted to relate to the mid-parental height centile. Length and weight may thus cross centiles over this initial period, depending on the disparity between the mother's and the father's height centiles, but from the age of 2 or 3, the child's height should have settled on the centile to which it should adhere until the age at which pubertal growth becomes relevant.

It is noteworthy that twins and higher multiples, who constitute about 2% of the population, are smaller than singletons at birth following comparable lengths of pregnancy, but frequently catch up postnatally.[10-12]

Box C indicates in a simplified way types of low birthweight infant, and the implications with regard to ongoing growth patterns sometimes provide a pointer to the aetiology underlying the smallness. The last group in the box, comprising those globally small infants with so-called "intrauterine growth retardation", includes many clinical types and causes, but the factors concerned are longstanding throughout the course of the pregnancy. Many conditions that have resulted in growth

---

Box C: Types of low birth weight infant

Weight in relation to gestational age	Clinical group	Prospects for subsequent growth
Appropriate	Preterm – short gestation	Good
Inappropriately light		
• Length affected less than weight	Short term adverse influence – undernutrition in late pregnancy (placental insufficiency)	Good
• Length and weight affected similarly	Long-term adverse influences – (from early in pregnancy)	Poor

---

retardation throughout pregnancy result in poor postnatal growth, and the status at birth is merely one point in an ongoing growth pattern. Such conditions include inherited pathological conditions affecting growth, and the sequelae to intrauterine infections.

Sometimes adverse effects on growth are primarily or partly due to chronic malnutrition of the developing fetus, which may be due to severe maternal undernutrition (perhaps secondary to chronic ill health) or to chronic placental insufficiency, et cetera. Excessive maternal use of drugs and similar substances, notably alcohol and tobacco, can have an irreversible adverse effect on the size of a baby. However, whether the cause of intrauterine growth retardation is known from the start, becomes evident after birth, or is never known, as a generalisation inappropriate low birth weight of this kind augurs badly for subsequent growth.

Maternal diabetes results in an adverse environment for the fetus which causes overgrowth, but postnatally, apart from the immediate consequences of insulin and glucose imbalance, the baby should grow and develop normally. In contrast, some inherent pathologies in a fetus may not result in an effect on growth at the time of birth because the optimal intrauterine environment of a healthy mother may prevent these manifestations in the fetus. Such conditions as congenital hypo-thyroidism or growth hormone deficiency will not usually be indicated by growth retardation until the postnatal period.

Nature of growth in infancy and early childhood

The pattern of growth antenatally and in the first 2–3 years of life is important, not only for its predictive value for long term subsequent growth but also because these are times in development which may set the stage for subsequent growth potential. Prolonged adverse influences on growth in the antenatal and postnatal periods may not subsequently be fully reversible, and the longer the adverse influence persists the worse the prognosis for growth. This effect is seen, for example, in such conditions as prolonged malabsorption, undernutrition, neglect, and social deprivation, which, though serious in their consequences at any age, are more likely to be reversible in terms of growth when occurring for the first time in older children.

Inheritance and familial factors

The predominant influence on growth within the overall population, accounting for most of the variations, is that of normal inheritance, primarily with regard to stature, but also in physique, degrees of fatness or thinness, and to a lesser extent timing of physical development (see Chapter 6). It is of primary importance to find out about these features in the parents and, if possible, siblings, in order to assess how likely it is that the growth pattern in a child that is causing concern can be attributed to inheritance (see Box D). Of course, though important, these are only components within an overall assessment, and if one parent is very tall and one very short any stature in a child could be explained depending on which parent he or she took after. It should be obvious that only the heights of the real parents and not step-parents are relevant! Occasionally the height of a parent may be shorter than it really should be because of injury or chronic disease.

In applying these guidelines it must be remembered that a few patho-logical conditions affecting growth may be dominantly inherited, in which circumstances 50% of the children would be expected to show the same growth problem as the affected parent. Such examples with short stature are achondroplasia and other bone dysplasias, Noonan's

---

Box D: How to evaluate the influence of parental height on that of a child

Child's expected height centile =

$$\frac{\text{Mother's height centile} + \text{Father's height centile}}{2}$$

or

Expected ultimate height of child when fully grown:

If a boy =

$$\frac{\text{Father's height} + (\text{Mother's height} + 5'' \, (12 \cdot 5 \text{ cm}))}{2}$$

If a girl =

$$\frac{(\text{Father's height} - 5'' \, (12 \cdot 5 \text{ cm})) + \text{Mother's height}}{2}$$

---

syndrome, and a few cases of congenital growth hormone deficiency. Marfan's syndrome is a dominantly inherited condition with tall stature.

Nutritional status

For satisfactory growth a child must be adequately nourished, having a food intake appropriate in both quality and quantity, and be able to assimilate that into body material following normal digestion and absorption. Undernutrition is likely to show its effect earlier and to a greater degree with regard to weight than length or height, as indicated by the position on centile charts. The evaluation of weight composition is considered in Chapter 4, and is fundamental to the diagnosis of causes of poor growth. The careful, thorough assessment of food intake by a dietitian should often be an early component of investigation, to find out whether a child's food intake is actually sufficient for normal growth. The development of anaemia, which is most commonly nutritional in origin, may have the ongoing effect of reducing appetite and perpetuating the problem.

General state of health

Almost all severe chronic illnesses will ultimately have an adverse effect on growth, and the presence of these should become evident by obtaining a good past history and from examination, for example chronic liver disease, chronic renal disease, and juvenile chronic arthritis. Some chronic diseases however – for example, chronic inflammatory bowel disease (Crohn's disease) or late presenting coeliac disease – may not have clinically obvious features yet may still have a severe adverse effect on growth. Growth retardation occurs in severe asthma as well as in other forms of severe atopy, and as it occurs in those who have never had corticosteroid treatment it is presumably related to the disease process itself, though sometimes it occurs through delayed puberty. The effect is frequently through reduced appetite and food intake, with the evidence of being underweight, but not necessarily so. Growth may be impaired by chronic hypoxia, as in severe pulmonary infections, upper airway obstruction (notably with sleep apnoea), or cyanotic heart disease. In illness weight can frequently be affected rapidly, but it must be sufficiently protracted to have a significant effect on height, particularly in prepubertal childhood when the expected height velocity is normally small (only about 5–6 cm a year), and it takes time for a fall-off to become evident. Unlike weight, which can fall, actual height once acquired is seldom lost in a child, and a fall-off in height velocity is unlikely to antedate the onset of the illness. The magnitude of the effect on growth is thus related to the duration of the illness. In certain circumstances, treatment (notably with high dose glucocorticosteroids) may be the cause of growth retardation rather than, or as much as, the illness itself. The degree to which subsequent catch up growth is possible will depend on many factors such as the duration and nature of the illness, the age period over which it occurred, the amount of potential growing time remaining, and the completeness of the cure.

Hormonal status

Many hormones are required for growth, and in healthy children these are produced in appropriate amounts. Only when their circulating levels are too low or too high for prolonged periods will there be an adverse effect on height. In hormonal imbalance weight is commonly affected in an opposite way to height, so that, with the exception of sex hormones,

---

Box E: Endocrine conditions causing short stature

Growth hormone
deficiency
Thyroid deficiency
Glucocorticoid excess
Sex hormones — deficiency or delay in production
causes short stature early
— excess or premature production
causes short stature ultimately
Diabetes mellitus — when control has been poor for a
long time

---

children with endocrine causes of short stature as shown in Box E tend to be overweight. In deficiencies of pituitary hormones, single or multiple hormones may be affected. Tall stature is a much less common cause of concern in childhood than short stature, and is seldom due to underlying pathology. Some endocrinological causes are listed in Box F.

Box F: Endocrine conditions causing tall stature

Growth hormone
excess (rare)
Thyrotoxicosis
Sex hormones — precocious production causes tall
stature early
— deficiency or extremely delayed
production may cause tall stature
ultimately (but not in Turner's
syndrome)

The effect of sex steroids on stature depends on the age at which they are active. Sex hormones, whether circulating as part of true puberty or for other pathological reasons, result in an initial acceleration of growth but subsequently cause cessation of growth when epiphyseal fusion ensues. Sexual development at a precocious age will therefore result in tallness at that time, but because growth also stops prematurely, ultimate stature is likely to be short. Conversely, when puberty with its associated growth spurt is delayed, stature will fall off compared with that of contemporaries, but growth may well continue to an older age and make up for the deficit, with a possible ultimate outcome of tall stature.

Psychological, psychosocial, and emotional aspects of growth

There is a clear relationship between psychological status and growth as well as with mental and intellectual development. The adverse effects on growth of severe psychological upset and emotional deprivation or long term abuse are well known. How this happens is not certain, sometimes being dependent on undernutrition, although sometimes there is a potentially reversible "switching off" of endocrine function. (Under such circumstances treatment with hormones would not be appropriate and probably not effective.) It is likely, however, that less extreme degrees of psychological disturbance may also affect growth in a less obvious, more subtle way, which may be difficult to recognise and more so to prove. Circumstances even occur when the adverse psychological effect of being small, particularly if associated with delay in puberty, may initiate a vicious circle of slowed growth and continuing delay.

Specific "syndromes" involving abnormalities of growth

The term "syndrome" is used of conditions, often with a characteristic physical appearance, in which there are many clinical features, of which abnormal growth is frequently one. Some of the commoner syndromes accounting for short stature are listed in Box G, and for tall stature in Box H. The short stature conditions, like many other "dysmorphic" conditions, have usually manifested intrauterine growth retardation, with inappropriately low birth weight as already discussed. Although endocrine deficiencies are not usually the cause of the poor growth, they can occasionally occur in some of these conditions, notably thyroid dysfunction in Down's syndrome or Turner's syndrome.

Basic abnormalities of bone growth, not due to endocrine or metabolic disease and frequently inherited, are bone dysplasias, the commonest being the dominantly inherited condition achondroplasia. This condition is clinically obvious, but there are many others in which a diagnosis is less apparent and the clue may lie in abnormal body proportions in

35

Box G: Commoner "syndromes" of short stature

Syndrome	Approximate incidence
Down's syndrome	1:700 births (increasing with maternal age – 1:1500 at 20; 1:100 at 40)
Silver–Russell syndrome	
Turner's syndrome	1:5000 births (1:2500 female births)
Noonan's syndrome	1:1000–1:2500 births
Fetal alcohol syndrome	
Prader–Willi syndrome	1:10 000 births
Congenital rubella	

Box H: Commoner "syndromes" of tall stature

Syndrome	Incidence
Klinefelter's syndrome (47,XXY karyotype)	1:500 male births
47,XYY karyotype	1:1000 male births
Marfan's syndrome	1:1000 births
Sotos syndrome (cerebral gigantism)	

---

which the limbs and spine are affected to differing degrees. Rickets is a condition of short stature (predominantly affecting the limbs) which is dependent on metabolic causation, being due to vitamin D deficiency or abnormality in its function.

4: Interpretation of weight

It is usually obvious from the first observation whether a child is fat or thin, but sometimes this initial opinion may be wrong and a more thorough evaluation is appropriate. A guide is provided in Box A. The first essential is to identify the child's weight centile position, which is usually what has triggered concern, frequently as the result of routine

---

Box A: How to evaluate weight

Relationship to height	Comparison of height and weight centile positions
Changes in weight with time	Serial observations of weight (and height) centiles and velocity centiles
Relation to pubertal status	Secondary sexual characteristics
Relative contributions of fatty and lean tissues	Skinfold measurements Mid-upper arm circumference
Skeletal proportions	Limb lengths compared to trunk length Body physique

---

measurements. But, although obvious, it is fundamental to recognise that *not all children who are above average weight are fat, and not all children who are below average weight are thin.*

Comparison of the weight centile position with that of the height is essential, and, as a generalisation, the weight centile for an individual should be matched fairly closely by the height centile. Such an observation is fundamental as the first point of evaluation and in the majority of cases this rule of thumb proves correct. However, *not all children whose weight is above average for height are fat*; they may have:

- Atypical body proportions – for example, trunk and head proportionately bigger than the limbs in length, girth, or both;
- Greater than average muscle (for example, athletes) and bone mass, with large body build;
- Puberty under way at an earlier than average age.

Also, *not all children whose weight is below average for height are thin*, they may have:

● Atypical body proportions – for example, limbs proportionately longer than the trunk;
● Less than average musculature, thin bones, and a slender physique;
● Delayed puberty.

As pointed out in Chapter 1, in the compilation of standard centiles the population, supposedly normal, was probably not optimal and contained an excess of overweight individuals so that in the upper centile range the "ideal" weight should probably be at a slightly lower centile than that for height.

In terms of their lengths, legs are lighter than trunk and head, hence the significance of the relative contribution of these to body weight in relation to overall height. Details of body proportions can be obtained by measurement of sitting height, derived leg lengths, and span, for which centile charts are available (see Chapter 2). Relationships of weight to height at an age when puberty becomes relevant are much harder to evaluate (see Chapter 6) and consideration of the stage of puberty is essential to interpretation and a better guideline than actual age.

Figure 4.1 illustrates very simply the great range in weight that may be found in normal prepubertal children of the same height and age.

Family growth pattern

Although sometimes variations in the weight/height relationships described above may be due to some underlying pathology, in the majority of cases these are normal variants. They frequently have an inherited basis, in terms of body build, degrees of fatness and thinness, timing of puberty, and body proportions. This is the most common explanation for disproportionately large or small heads, or atypical limb/trunk ratios and can be identified from similar observations on one or both parents. Usually this indicates that an underlying pathology is unlikely, although occasionally pathological conditions affecting these aspects are dominantly inherited (for example, bone dysplasias).

Body mass index (BMI)

In adults this index, which is weight (in kilograms) divided by the square of height (in metres) (W/H^2) is frequently used as an indication

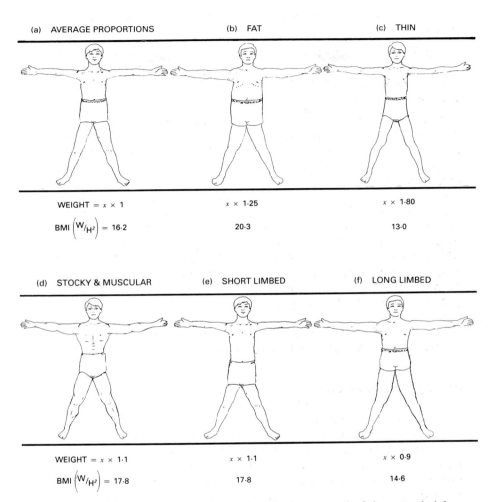

(a) AVERAGE PROPORTIONS   (b) FAT   (c) THIN

| WEIGHT $= x \times 1$ | $x \times 1.25$ | $x \times 1.80$ |
| BMI $\left(W/H^2\right) = 16.2$ | 20.3 | 13.0 |

(d) STOCKY & MUSCULAR   (e) SHORT LIMBED   (f) LONG LIMBED

| WEIGHT $= x \times 1.1$ | $x \times 1.1$ | $x \times 0.9$ |
| BMI $\left(W/H^2\right) = 17.8$ | 17.8 | 14.6 |

Figure 4.1   Normal prepubertal boys aged 10 years and of the same height

of an individual's fatness or thinness. Although some of the factors just described may influence this as well, it is nevertheless quite a useful guideline. In children, however, it is of no value. The index increases progressively through the years of puberty (Figure 4.2) and could only be meaningful if compared with average values for the same age or stage of pubertal development. This is clearly impractical, and even with this common parameter, the range in normal individuals of the same degree

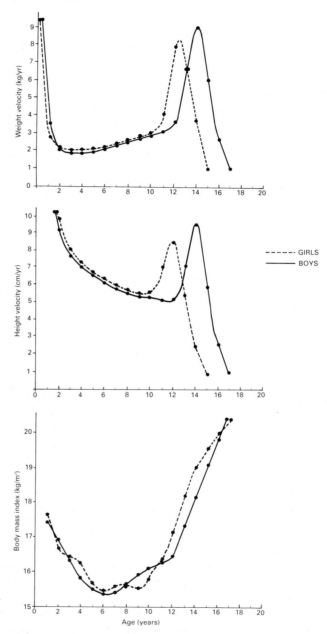

Figure 4.2   Mean weight velocity, height velocity, and body mass index through childhood

of fatness will be considerable (Figure 4.1). The same comments apply to the inappropriateness of the use of weight to height ratios.

Changes in weight

True height changes, as distinct from misleading changes dependent on technique or timing, are only realistically evident over periods of 3 months or more (except at puberty). Weight, however, can change dramatically over days, or even hours, particularly in circumstances of illness, but also in the normal course of events, dependent on intake of food and drink and loss in terms of excretion of faeces, urine, or sweat. Unlike height velocity charts, weight charts allow for the possibility of a negative velocity.

How to evaluate weight changes

Several questions must be asked when evaluating weight changes. Are they appropriate for age? Are they appropriate for height changes? Are they appropriate for pubertal status? Do they reflect appropriate changes in fat and lean body mass?

Whether or not weight changes are appropriate and match height changes will be evident from the use of centile charts in the years before puberty. Figure 4.2 shows that weight velocities fall dramatically during the first 2 years of life and are only of the order of 2 kg per year for boys and girls from age 2 to 5. Weight velocity then increases, but only gradually, prior to the dramatic rise at puberty. In contrast, height velocity falls progressively through childhood to the lowest value of about 5 cm per year just before puberty. However, the enormous normal variation in the age of puberty makes evaluation then much more difficult. The different patterns of growth to be expected at puberty in relation to its timing are illustrated in Figure 4.3. The proportionate fall off from the average in late developers appears much greater in terms of weight than height, and similarly the gains in early developers. This is discussed more fully in Chapter 6. The massive weight gain at puberty is predominantly lean body mass and not fat. To evaluate whether weight changes are due to fat, or muscle and other lean tissues, is important both in normal development and in situations of disease and its treatment, and the easiest method is by the use of skinfold calipers, which will show serial changes in subcutaneous fat – a good index of overall body fat. These will demonstrate, for example, that the massive weight gain at the peak of adolescent growth in boys is usually accompanied by a fall in fat measurements, and similar findings of fat

41

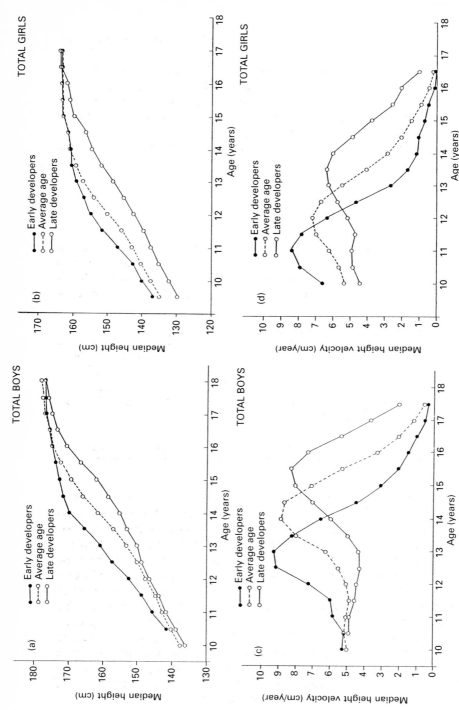

Figure 4.3 Height (median) division based on timing of puberty for (a) boys and (b) girls; height velocity (median) division based on timing of puberty for (c) boys and (d) girls

42

reduction often accompany the dramatic early increases in weight in response to treatment of growth hormone deficiency or hypothyroidism. Such information is particularly important in evaluating changes in fat composition in the treatment of obese adolescents, in whom a weight increase may well be appropriate and desirable as long as it is due to the "normal" gain of lean body mass and accompanied by a fall in fat.

Obesity

This is very common in childhood, and in the majority is not due to underlying pathology. Obesity commonly shows a familial pattern, and it is said that if one parent is obese there is a 40–50% chance that a child will be also, and if both parents are obese a 70–80% chance –

Table 4.1 Types of obesity in the growing child

	Cause	Stature	Physiological age (bone age and puberty)	Incidence	Family history
Exogenous	Non-pathological (food intake excessive for amount of energy used)	Tall	Advanced	Common	Common
Endogenous	Underlying pathology	Short	Retarded	Rare	Rare

and also probably the family pets! Table 4.1 indicates the pointers in distinguishing these exogenously obese children from the less than 10% in which there is a recognisable underlying pathology (illustrated by Figure 4.4). During the growing years exogenously obese children are usually big in all proportions, being taller (than expectation on the basis of mid-parental centile) and with increased bony proportions and often muscle. Clearly the amount of fat is greatly in excess of these other components or the individuals would not be considered obese. This does not imply that they will end up taller as adults, for during their growing years they are frequently physically advanced, which probably accounts for their taller stature, with advanced skeletal ages, and often go into puberty earlier than average, but with the consequence that they reach their full stature earlier too (Figure 4.5). In that minority of children in whom there is an underlying pathological cause for the

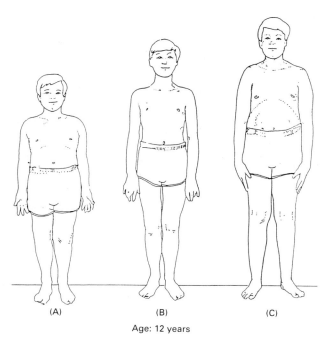

Age: 12 years

Figure 4.4   The relationship of growth in height to growth in weight in different types of overweight (A) endogenous pathological and (C) exogenous compared with (B) lean normal

obesity, they are usually short of stature and often physiologically delayed. Clearly treatment in this group must be primarily directed at this underlying pathology where possible, and success is unlikely with the basic dietary measures alone which form the primary approach to treatment of the exogenously obese children.

There are many pathologies associated with overweight, though most are uncommon, and the more familiar ones are listed in Box B and illustrated later (Chapter 10). In some syndromes obesity is a cardinal feature, but in other syndromes of short stature, such as Down's syndrome and Turner's syndrome, a proportion will be obese (as will be a proportion of the overall normal population), but obesity is not a component of the syndrome as such and many are not overweight. Children suffering from conditions associated with unavoidable inactivity, such as neurological, muscular, and orthopaedic conditions, will frequently become obese.

44

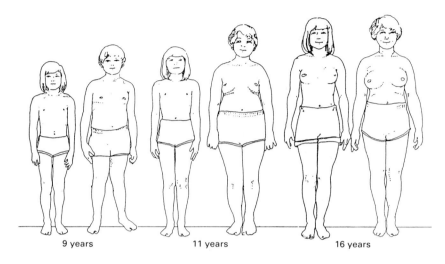

Figure 4.5 The growth pattern of two healthy girls, one lean and one fat, through the teenage years

---

Box B: Causes of endogenous obesity

Endocrine	• Acquired hypothyroidism
	• Growth hormone deficiency (isolated or as a component of hypopituitarism)
	• Glucocorticoid excess (endogenous or as the result of treatment)
	• Hyperinsulinism (not short stature) (usually overtreatment of diabetes)
Syndromes (rare)	• Prader–Willi
	• Laurence–Moon–Biedl
	• In a proportion of children with short stature "syndromes", for example, Down's, Turner's

The role of the dietitian

The dietitian is invaluable, not only in the obvious advice essential for treatment, but also in assessing the actual food intake. It is difficult to evaluate, on the basis of a history taken in a hurried clinic or surgery, whether the reported food intake is likely to be correct and is reasonable and appropriate in quantity and quality. The dietitian can evaluate this much more precisely and answer what is often the first question: Is this child having a food intake which is sufficient and appropriate for normal growth at this age, or one which is in excess of the needs of an average child of this age? The approach to underweight children is different if it is known that they are not actually taking in enough food to supply the needs for growth than if they are having an adequate intake. Likewise, if it is obvious that a child is overeating, dietary advice will be easier to give, though not necessarily easy to implement! It is, of course, evident that the requirements of children of the same age vary greatly even within a family and the food intake of one fat child and one thin child may be the same, and presumably the explanation lies in the different degrees of energy expenditure. What is really happening in the home and at school and in between with regard to eating and drinking is very difficult to document, and the dietitian can usually only interpret what is actually said. Sometimes a health visitor, district nurse, or social worker may be the person to visit the home to make direct observations and offer advice (see Chapter 9).

5: Physiological and skeletal age

Healthy children of the same sex and calendar age show a great range in their level of physical development. Over the age range at which the changes of puberty are likely to occur this variation becomes obvious, but prior to this, on basic examination, there is little if any indication as to whether an individual is average in the state of development, advanced, or retarded compared with the average. A simple method of identifying this state of development is, however, through the radiological estimation of skeletal age (bone age). Intellectual or mental development, though possibly showing a slight trend in variation in timing in the same direction as that of physical development, by no means parallels it, and the magnitude of the variation in terms of rates of intellectual maturity is not nearly so great.

This variation in the state of physical development at any particular age has considerable implications with regard to differences of growth potential, and although, in practice, skeletal age estimations are not often undertaken outside the hospital setting, an awareness of the significance of this factor in the interpretation of growth is of value, particularly so at the ages when the consideration of pubertal status becomes relevant.

Skeletal age

Although other methods have been advocated, the best and simplest depend on radiographs of the wrist and hand. A popular method involves comparing the appearance of these radiographs with standards to which have been attributed ages of bone development for an average individual. The most widely used system of this kind, that of Greulich and Pyle,[13] is quick and relatively simple, but it is approximate and based on American standards which are not appropriate for British and European populations. When this technique is applied with consideration of the status of individual bones, as in the originally described method, more precise answers can be obtained, but in practice comparison of radiographic appearance is usually more casual and inevitably imprecise, and difficulties arise when individual bones are not developing at similar rates.

47

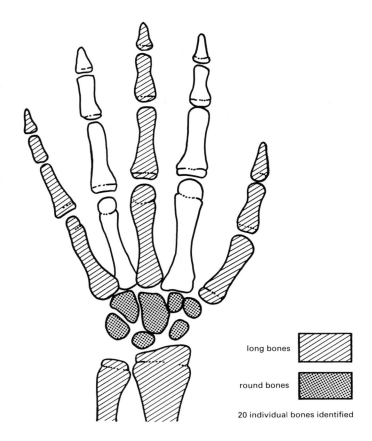

long bones	
round bones	
20 individual bones identified	

Figure 5.1 Bones of wrist and hand incorporated in TW2 assessments

A more accurate method, appropriate for European populations, is the TW2 method devised by Tanner and colleagues.[14] In this a score is worked out for the state of development of 20 bones of the wrist and hand – eight "carpal" (round) bones (wrist) and 12 "long" bones (the lower radius and ulna, metacarpals, and phalanges) (Figure 5.1). These values are totalled to provide a skeletal score for which a "skeletal age" can be directly read from tables. Evaluation does not depend on the size of the bones as such, for hands with bones of very different sizes may have the same bone age, but on the presence of the bones and epiphyses and the relationship of their size, shape, and markings, and ultimately the degree of fusion of the epiphyses to the shafts of the long bones.

These methods can only be used when the appearances of the bones are basically normal, and cannot be realistically evaluated when bones are deformed or damaged as in the more gross bone dysplasias, severe metabolic upsets, or arthritic conditions affecting the hands. The radiographs should be taken by experienced radiographers with correct positioning of the hands and accurate exposure. Interpretation is somewhat subjective, even with experienced observers, but reported changes in bone age over the course of time become more meaningful when the radiographs are read by the same person.

The usefulness of bone age estimations

The ways in which bone ages may be of value are indicated in Box A.

Box A: Uses of bone age estimations

In diagnosis of:

• Conditions with short stature

• Conditions with tall stature

In predicting growth potential and ultimate height

In monitoring treatment

The dividing line between the degree of retardation or advancement of bone age that can be attributed to physiological variation and that which occurs in pathological conditions cannot be precisely defined. This radiological investigation is merely one tool within an overall assessment and should seldom be interpreted in isolation. Physiological normal variation can be considerable, and Figure 5.2 shows the bony appearances of the hands of four healthy 14 year old boys with bone ages ranging from 12 to 16 years, the lowest being in a completely prepubertal boy and the greatest in one of almost adult maturity.

A rough guide to show how pathological conditions may affect bone age is shown in Box B. The degree of the effect in any condition is, however, considerable – depending on the duration of the illness and

49

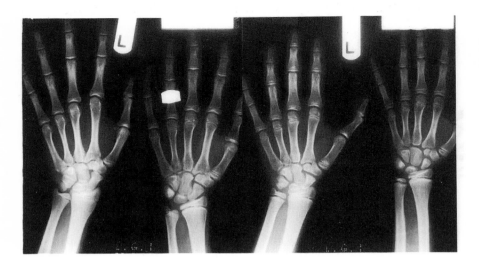

Figure 5.2   Radiographs of four normal 14 year old boys

its severity. It is important to recognise that if bone age is affected by a disorder, the degree of that effect cannot be greater than the length of time over which the illness has been present. The degree of retardation of bone age is an indication of the theoretical extra residual growth, as this reflects the years of growth remaining to bony maturity better than does chronological age. However, this requires a situation in which this growth potential can be achieved – and this is usually the outcome in circumstances where the deviation in bone age is physiological. An example illustrating the height difference that might be expected at maturity in healthy normal boys and girls of the same height at the same age but with a range of different bone ages is shown in Table 5.1. These estimates, based on the standard method of prediction,[14] are very approximate, depending on the state of pubertal development, but do give some indication of the possible range.

Where the underlying cause of abnormal growth and bone age is pathological, appropriate treatment will be required for improvement in growth. There must also be sufficient time available, for in older individuals the time for residual growth is limited when puberty occurs.

The pathological conditions which affect bone age most strikingly are endocrine (as shown in Box B), thyroid conditions being the most dramatic of all. Hypothyroidism is probably the only condition which

50

Box B: How disease and illness may affect bone age

Bone age	*Indications*
Markedly retarded	Longstanding endocrine deficiencies (thyroid, growth hormone, hypopituitarism) Failure of puberty (sex hormone deficiencies)
Moderately retarded	Chronic disease (nutritional, malabsorption, metabolic, infections). Psychosocial deprivation
Close to normal	Dysmorphic conditions, intrauterine growth retardation, non-endocrine "syndromes" affecting growth; bone dysplasias
Moderately advanced	(Exogenous obesity) Sexual precocity
Markedly advanced	Thyrotoxicosis

Table 5.1 Variation in height predictions resulting from differences in bone age in healthy 12 year old boys and 10 year old girls of average height

	Bone age (years)	Average predicted adult height (cm)
Boys	(12 years old; 147 cm tall)	
	9	183·0
	10	180·4
	11	177·8
	12	175·2
	13	172·6
	14	170·0
	15	167·4
Girls	(10 years old; 136 cm tall)	
	7	172·6
	8	169·4
	9	166·2
	10	163·0
	11	159·8
	12	156·6
	13	153·4

51

retards bone age to a greater extent than it affects height (which effect is in itself extreme), though this does not mean, as one might infer from the above discussion, that treated individuals will end up taller than they would have done if they had never been hypothyroid. Conversely, the dramatic advancement of bone age, which exceeds the associated acceleration in height in hyperthyroidism, does not usually have an adverse effect on ultimate height in individuals who are appropriately treated. It is thus impossible to generalise with regard to height prognoses following treatment in those pathological situations which affect bone age, and height predictions based on standard methods appropriate for "normals" are unreliable. The outcome for height depends on many factors, notably the appropriateness of treatment and the age of the individual at the time of its initiation. Bone age advancement resulting from sexual precocity or inappropriate use of androgens or oestrogens is the most obvious circumstance to result in reduction of growth potential and adult stature.

The change in bone age through the course of long term treatment is one aspect that aids in the management. If dosage is incorrect, growth advancement may be slower than bone age advancement, thus losing the benefit of the theoretical extra potential. Ideally, the bone age should not advance at a faster rate than the height age, if optimal height is to be achieved in short stature conditions with retarded bone age, and conversely, in situations with pathologically advanced bone ages, treatment should be accompanied by a reduction in the degree of bone age advancement. (Occasionally conditions of unacceptably tall stature are deliberately treated with high doses of sex hormones in order to advance bone age rapidly and reduce ultimate height.)

In normal circumstances, in healthy children, the bone age advances year by year approximately in parallel with actual age advancement. This is not so, however, at the time of puberty, for at the age of most rapid growth in height, bone age also advances more rapidly than the previous "one year of bone age per one year of chronological age." In delayed puberty the rate of bone age advancement is slowed down, and in puberty which occurs at an early age bone age advancement occurs earlier (see Figure 5.3). There comes an age, of course, when no further growth is possible, and this is indicated radiologically by fusion of the epiphyses to the shafts of the bones. This is the consequence of puberty and will not occur without puberty. Puberty has a twofold effect on growth – initially speeding it up, but subsequently stopping it. Growth potential and the pattern of growth are not essentially linked with

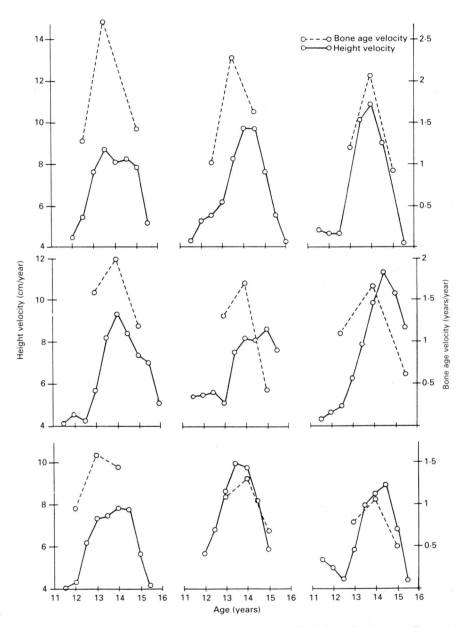

Figure 5.3 Comparison of bone age velocity and height velocity at puberty in 9 normal boys

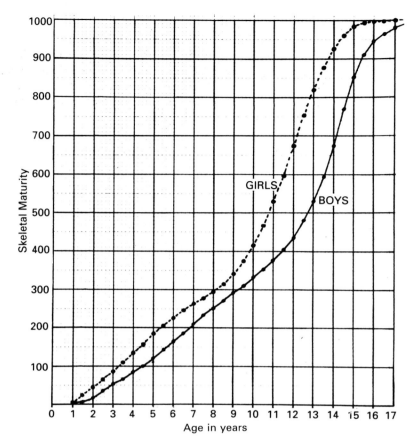

Figure 5.4   Median bone age in relation to skeletal score (TW2 method) for boys and girls

reaching a certain chronological age, but to the pubertal status at that age. *If puberty is well advanced, the radiological demonstration that bony epiphyses are fused to the shafts proves conclusively that no further growth is possible, whatever the age.*

Girls enter puberty two years earlier on average than boys, reach their age of most rapid growth two years earlier, and reach full adult height likewise. Not surprisingly, therefore, their bony development is about two years earlier throughout, but what is surprising, perhaps, is that this difference in bone development is evident through the full course of childhood, including the younger ages when the heights and weights of girls and boys and their basic hormonal status are very similar (Figure 5.4).

54

Dental development

There is no close relationship between dental maturity and skeletal maturity, though the overall trend in timing is similar. Early developing children tend to erupt their teeth earlier, and girls earlier than boys, but precise observations on dental development are not helpful with regard to assessment of overall growth.

6: Puberty

Growth changes are so dramatic and fundamental at puberty that, within the wide age range when puberty could conceivably be occurring, it is essential to assess the pubertal status. Without that knowledge, interpretation of the significance of retardation of height and weight may be incorrect. Likewise, in a situation where growth speeds up unexpectedly, it is important to check whether or not this is due to sexual development.

It is difficult to describe or define normal puberty, because of the enormous variation within a healthy population in the timing, sequence, and magnitude of the changes.

Boys

The first sign of puberty in the vast majority of boys is growth of the testes. This is a sign that is seldom looked for but it is a very important one, for if such growth is observed it gives good grounds for anticipating that puberty proper, in the layman's sense of the term, will be following, including the associated growth package. There may be quite a long interval, up to a year or so, before anything dramatic occurs, and two years before the age of most rapid growth (peak height velocity), but nevertheless these *will* happen. Without this sign one is not in a position to predict the timing of onset of puberty clinically. The prepubertal testis is small and changes little in size over the years (volume about 1 ml or the size of a plum stone). At the onset of puberty testicular growth is rapid and, arbitrarily, a size of 4 ml is considered in the Tanner staging to be Stage 2 or the entry into puberty. Testicular size can be estimated precisely with the use of an orchidometer (Figure 6.1), but this is usually unnecessary as the change is obvious if looked for. The adult testis measures 20 ml on average, but with a range of 15 to 25 ml. The sequence of events is very variable, except that the age of peak growth rate is relatively late when genital development, and usually pubic hair, is well advanced. On average breaking of the voice occurs close to the age of rapid growth, but is usually a gradual process. Axillary hair seldom appears until pubic hair is well developed, and the appearance of facial hair is later, so that when a young man needs to shave regularly he is usually effectively fully grown (Figure 6.2).

The secondary sexual clinical features of puberty in boys are essentially the result of the progressively increasing levels of circulating testosterone

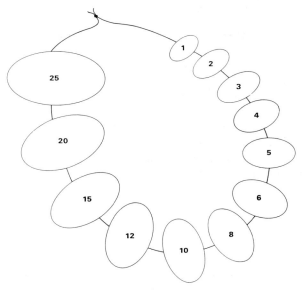

Figure 6.1   Orchidometer (figures indicate the volume of the testis in ml)

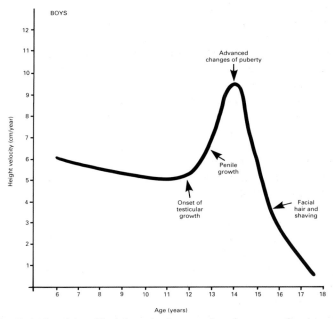

Figure 6.2   Relationship of height velocity to other features of puberty in boys (average ages)

from the developing testes. Initially these increasing levels accelerate growth but presumably, ultimately, above a certain level, they cause its cessation by fusing epiphyses. (This explanation is somewhat simplistic as there are also changes in other growth related hormones at puberty, notably growth hormone.) There is also increased production of adrenal androgens in the course of normal "physiological" puberty, which are of far less potency than testosterone and contribute little to the overall picture. Occasionally, however, the timing of onset of "adrenarche" is before gonadal activity, and pubic hair may develop sparsely as the first feature, without the gonadal component of true puberty; this usually follows soon, but until there is testicular growth it cannot be guaranteed.

Girls

The changes of puberty are on average two years earlier in girls than in boys, and the sequence of events is variable also. In over three quarters of girls the first feature of puberty is breast budding, and the speed up of growth occurs at an early stage (Figure 6.3). In a significant minority of normal girls, however, pubic hair is the first feature, either alone or synchronously with breast development. Onset of menstruation is almost always a late feature, invariably following the age of most rapid growth, and only a small proportion of the total growth of puberty occurs after the menarche. High levels of circulating oestrogens ultimately fuse the epiphyses. As with boys, there is an adrenal component to puberty and some of the features of puberty, such as pubic hair, are dependent on androgens derived from the adrenal, which may account for these features sometimes being the first. Though ovarian activity usually follows soon, there is no guarantee that it will in pathological situations.

The growth of healthy boys and girls who develop earlier or later than average

At whatever age puberty occurs, the growth "package" is essentially similar, with an onset following the gradual decline in height velocity through childhood. This package comprises an acceleration to a peak velocity followed by the decline to ultimate cessation of growth – a

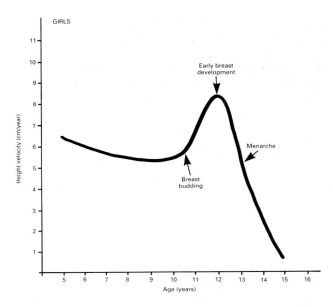

Figure 6.3   Relationship of height velocity to other features of puberty in girls (average ages)

process which averages five years in duration. If the age range of onset is within one to two years of the average age, the difference in the magnitude of the peak compensates for the variable duration of pre-pubertal growth on which this pubertal "package" is superimposed (see Figure 4.3). When the deviation in timing is larger, however, this compensation is incomplete, and precocious developers are likely to end up shorter in stature and late developers taller than would otherwise have been anticipated. Figure 6.4 compares data from a personal study of the growth of 100 schoolgirls and 200 schoolboys on the timing and magnitude of components of certain features of growth of early, average aged, and late developing boys and girls.[5]

The height of early developing boys and girls will deviate upwards from their previous height centile line as they leave their contemporaries behind, but the earlier slow down and completion of growth will bring them ultimately close to their original centiles. This pattern of growth is a cause of concern in children who are tall initially – notably girls and commonly on a familial basis. If the accelerating growth and worrying tallness at that early age can be linked with the pubertal process,

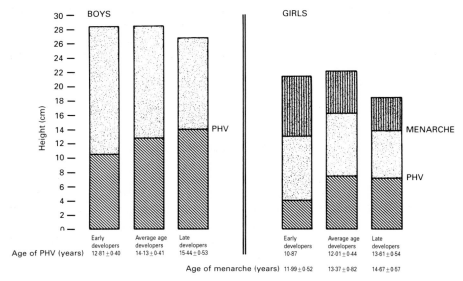

Figure 6.4 Height increments associated with puberty for early, average aged and late developing boys and girls

assurance that ultimate stature will not be unacceptably tall is often appropriate, and particularly if a girl has reached the menarche, following which there is usually little residual growth.

The converse problem is particularly common with healthy, short stature children, notably boys, who are delayed in puberty. Here, height falls off from the previous centile which, if low already, results in their degree of shortness becoming more marked, and causes considerable embarrassment and emotional upset, particularly as it is linked with sexual immaturity. Reassurance can be given regarding ultimate height as there is considerable extra growth potential compared with the average child of the same age. However, the immediate concerns need considerable support and understanding to help cope with the psychological stresses. Predicting when puberty will happen is not possible until the first clinical features are evident (though the degree of bone age retardation may be helpful), but when these features do appear, most commonly breast budding in girls and testicular growth in boys, confident reassurance can be given. The height of the girls will accelerate within the next few months and peak about a year later. Progress with boys will, however, be slower. It will probably be over a year before any dramatic changes follow this initial feature and two years or more before the age of maximal growth rate, and continuing psychological support may be needed. If the delay and emotional distress become extreme, these may be grounds for speeding up the progression of early puberty with gonadotrophin or sex hormone treatment, and this is considered in Chapter 9. These different growth patterns for early and late developing boys and girls are illustrated in Figure 4.3 (p. 42).

Factors influencing the timing of puberty

There are many factors within the healthy population that appear to influence the timing of puberty, many of which are interrelated (see Box A). Social factors probably link with nutrition as well as basic health standards. In general, well off populations enter puberty earlier than the poor, and urban populations earlier than rural. The effects of nutrition on growth seem to have a greater lasting impact before puberty, for

---

Box A: Non-pathological factors relating to the timing of puberty

Sex	Girls earlier than boys
Nutrition	Undernourished and thin later than well nourished and fat
Familial	
Racial	
Stress – psychological	Delays puberty
Secular trend	Puberty has become earlier through the years
Physical activity	Extreme competitive sports delay puberty
Light–darkness rhythms	Blind children develop earlier
Altitude	Later at high altitudes
Social factors	Later in the underprivileged

---

though puberty is delayed in the undernourished, the actual increase in height through the course of puberty is changed little. Thin and short individuals tend to go into puberty later than those who are fat and tall.

Racial trends are difficult to explain, do not seem primarily to be climatic, and may be dependent on other environmental variables influencing general health and wellbeing.

There is a definite familial factor in the timing of puberty, which can be reassuring in circumstances where marked advancement or delay can be linked to a similar pattern in one or both parents and other members of the family. Adults may find it difficult to recollect the age at which they passed through puberty, though many women will know the age of their own menarche, which is a good indicator of the timing of puberty as a whole, but men have no such equivalent marker.

It is not clear why extreme competitive physical activity delays puberty, but this is well documented, particularly in girls, in whom the age of menarche can be markedly retarded. Participants in gymnastics, ballet dancing, and running activities show this effect, though seldom, curiously, competitive swimmers.

An advancement in the age of puberty, as best evidenced by the age of menarche, has occurred over the last century in many countries, although in most it now appears to have halted. Undoubtedly improved nutrition and general health have contributed to this, but cannot fully explain the trend. The state of health is a powerful influence both in individuals and within communities, and chronic illness of many kinds, with or without undernutrition, delays puberty.

Precocious sexual development

Changes in growth, as indicated, are so closely related to sexual development that abnormalities in the pubertal process are fundamental with regard to growth. Sexual development occurring inappropriately early may represent true "central" precocious puberty, with features typical of normal puberty but occurring very early, in which case the normal sequence of the pubertal process is to be expected early, or it may represent some limited form of sexual development dependent on inappropriate sex hormone production or tissue responsiveness, not the result of central gonadotrophin drive. The age at which puberty should be considered as abnormally early or outside the "physiological" age range is very arbitrary, but, as a guideline, features appearing before the

---

Box B: Concerns raised by precocious sexual development

- That there may be a sinister underlying cause
- That it is psychologically unacceptable:
  embarrassment of inappropriately early sexual changes,
  excessively tall stature, and early onset of menstruation in
  girls, vulnerability of young girls
- That there will be long term sequelae – in fact, the only one is
  short stature

---

age of 8 in girls or 9 in boys may be considered a cause for concern. The concerns which may be aroused are indicated in Box B.

True precocious puberty is much commoner in girls than in boys, and in the majority of cases in girls it is idiopathic, that is, without recognisable underlying pathology. There is commonly a similar history in a parent, which is further reassurance that it is benign. In boys puberty occurring unequivocally early is uncommon, and in over half the cases is due to an underlying central nervous system pathology which must be looked for. The psychological and social implications of precocious puberty are considerable, including those related to growth. As already indicated, the acceleration of growth may result in conspicuous tallness compared with peers at the time, but subsequent premature cessation of growth may well result in short stature — of increasing likelihood the younger the age at which puberty develops and if the preceding stature was short anyway.

If the full picture of puberty does not develop, the condition is probably not true puberty. Sometimes, in girls, isolated early breast development may occur — premature thelarche – most commonly in the 2–3 year old girl, but this is benign, regresses spontaneously, and is not accompanied by speed up of growth or bone age. Occasionally isolated androgenic activity manifests itself as pubic hair, or growth of the clitoris, or both, and though this may be benign it needs investigation and may be associated with accelerated growth.

In boys the clue to whether or not precocious sexual development is true puberty (that is, central) is the observation of testicular size. The first feature of true puberty is usually growth of the testes, but if these are still infantile in size the probability is that the source of androgens is not testicular (and is most likely adrenal). Almost all the clinical features of puberty in boys are the result of androgen production (testosterone in true puberty) but an identical clinical picture will be seen if excess androgen production is adrenal in origin, except that the testicles will remain small. In either case growth will be excessive initially, but with the long term consequence of short stature due to premature epiphyseal fusion.

Extreme delay of sexual development

The age at which delayed puberty will arouse concern is, like precocious puberty, arbitrary. On purely clinical grounds, in the absence of other suspicious features in an otherwise healthy child, one need not be concerned by the complete absence of signs of puberty at ages less than 14 in girls or 16 in boys, although the presence of clinical abnormalities, notably excessive thinness, would cause concern earlier (for example, anorexia, malabsorption, Crohn's disease, or asthma). However, this is usually not the criterion that initiates action, but rather the concern expressed by the child himself or herself or the family, or the comments of other people, usually resulting from an awareness of the growth failure and the increasingly evident short stature. Teasing and bullying at school may be a great burden, particularly for boys, and evaluation and investigation of the clinical problem, and possibly treatment, would then be required. The implications of delayed puberty are indicated in the Box C.

Box C: Concerns raised by delayed or incomplete sexual development

- That there may be a sinister underlying cause

- That puberty will never occur

- The emotional and psychological upset of immaturity (particularly when associated with short stature)

- That there will be long term sequelae

In lay terminology puberty in girls and menarche are often not distinguished. Clinically, however, it makes a great difference whether delay in menarche is the expected consequence of delayed puberty as a whole, in which case no speed up of growth will have occurred and it is the puberty as such that warrants assessment, or that menstruation has not occurred in a girl who has reached a sufficiently advanced state of development for it to be expected and who is almost fully grown. In that circumstance attention should be directed to anatomical causes, or polycystic ovarian disease.

In the majority of cases, as already indicated, delay in puberty in otherwise healthy children is physiological, particularly if there is a family history and the child is thin. Evidence of testicular growth in boys, a sign not normally noticed, or the beginnings of breast development in girls, indicates that puberty is under way. Most children with extreme delay in puberty will be investigated in time, and if necessary treated, but if nothing is done growth will continue at a slow steady prepubertal rate for a very long time as the sex hormones that fuse epiphyses are not present. Thus height may for a period be short due to the absence of the normal growth spurt, but ultimately the continuing growth will result in tall (usually proportionately long limbed) stature. If stature remains short with advancing age, this may point to an underlying endocrine dysfunction, or Turner's syndrome in girls – who remain short of stature even if treated with oestrogens to bring on puberty. In any girl with unexplained short stature and delayed puberty, even in the absence of the classical features of Turner's syndrome, this diagnosis should be considered (see Chapter 10).

When it comes to investigation of delayed puberty, this will usually be conducted in hospital, but the first simple investigation will be an estimation of blood gonadotrophin levels, which will distinguish whether the problem is gonadal (in which case gonadotrophins will be high) or at the hypothalamic–pituitary level (with low gonadotrophins) with potentially normal but unstimulated gonads. Unfortunately, there is no simple way of distinguishing those causes of hypothalamic–pituitary failure that are due to an underlying pathology from those that are due to physiological delay, and this may well have to await resolution with time. Endocrine causes of pubertal delay are usually linked with overweight, and such individuals are not thin, as are the majority of children with delayed puberty, and may well warrant earlier referral. In delayed puberty low grade adrenal activity may be evidenced by the presence of sparse pubic hair as an isolated feature of sexual development, but on its own this is not an indication of puberty as such and may well occur in situations of gonadal failure.

The interrelationships of growth with puberty are complex but always relevant and of great significance.

7: Pointers towards diagnosis of abnormal growth

Previous chapters have discussed the range of growth patterns that can occur in "normal" and "abnormal" circumstances. In this chapter these are brought together to provide a simple framework on which growth problems can be evaluated. Table 7.1 summarises the aspects of growth that should be considered in order to ascertain the likelihood that growth is abnormal, and therefore justify follow up and investigation, and in the very broadest way provides pointers to the type of pathology that might be involved. The relevant chapters in which these aspects are individually considered are indicated in the table. Specific conditions of abnormal growth are discussed in Chapter 10.

Features 1–3 of Table 7.1 provide the basis for referral (see Chapter 2), but do not necessarily in themselves provide sufficient information to point to specific diagnostic groups of growth problems. Further evidence for this is provided by features 4–8.

Weight–height relationships

Weight centile greater than height

This is most commonly due to obesity, the causes of which, endogenous and exogenous, are discussed in Chapter 4, p. 43. The chapter, however, also indicates that there are other reasons why weight and height centiles may not match up.

Weight centiles less than height

It is important to recognise that loss of weight can occur quickly in acute illnesses, due either to loss of appetite, or to increased losses through vomiting, diarrhoea, sweating, and so on. These transient conditions are usually easily distinguished from those where there is a long term state of being underweight. The latter usually result in a

Table 7.1   Guidelines for identification of abnormal growth

Feature	Causes for concern	Reference
1 Height centile position	Concern proportional to degree of deviation from the mean	Table 2.4 (p. 26)
2 Height velocity centile	Velocity over the course of a year below 25th centile or above 75th centile	Table 1.2 (p. 6) Table 2.4 (p. 26)
3 Comparison with height centile of parents and siblings	Concern proportional to degree of deviation from mid-parental centile (and siblings' centiles), but there may be inherited growth problems	Table 2.4 (p. 26) Chapter 3, Box D (p. 32)
4 Comparison of weight and height (and head circumference) positions	Marked disparity Clue to possible type of pathology	(p. 27) (pp. 37, 43)
5 Abnormal appearance		
a Abnormal body proportion	Great deviation in ratio of limb to trunk length	Table 2.3 (p. 22)
b Other abnormal feature (or intellectual deficit) "syndromes"	Diagnostic clinical features	Chapter 3, Boxes G and H (p. 36)
6 Inappropriate size at birth	Outlying position on birth weight for gestational age centiles	Chapter 3, Box C (p. 30)
7 Atypical pattern of sexual development (physiological or pathological)	Atypical growth linked with inappropriate age of sexual development	Fig. 4.3 (p. 42)
a Precocious	Tall early, short ultimately	Chapter 3, Boxes E and F (p. 34)
b Extreme delay	Short early, may become tall ultimately	Chapter 3, Boxes E and F (p. 34)
8 Chronic ill health or deprivation	Chronic symptoms and physical signs linked with poor growth	(p. 33)

subsequent slowing down of growth in stature, except in some hypermetabolic states such as thyrotoxicosis. A basic approach is suggested in Box A.

Box A: Causes of long term underweight

Normal variations of physique, muscularity, and body build (see pp. 37–38)

Abnormal health	Commoner underlying causes
INADEQUATE FOOD INTAKE	
Too little food offered	Poverty, neglect, ignorance
Poor appetite	Many chronic illnesses – for example, metabolic, acidosis, anoxia, infections, malignancies, etc.
	Anorexia nervosa – psychological causes
	Anaemia – notably iron deficiency
Difficulties in swallowing	Anatomical and obstructive causes
	Neurological causes
	Breathing difficulties, for example, upper airways obstruction
	Breathlessness and fatigue with heart failure or severe respiratory conditions
INCREASED LOSSES	
Vomiting	Many chronic illnesses, for example, metabolic, acidosis, infections, raised intracranial pressure
	Bulimia
Increased faecal loss	Chronic bowel infections – parasites (for example, giardiasis)
	Malabsorptive states – coeliac disease, cystic fibrosis, food intolerances
Polyuria	Diabetes – mellitus or insipidus
INCREASED METABOLISM	Thyrotoxicosis (tall stature)
	Diabetes mellitus
	Chronic infections
	Malignancies

If a disease process is suspected, the initial question is whether the food intake is actually sufficient for the child's requirements for growth. If not, then why not? There are many reasons for a poor appetite, as indicated, but it is worth noting that it may be due to anaemia, and occasionally chronic upper airway obstruction, for example, due to blocked nose or enlarged adenoids, which may make eating difficult. A dramatic improvement may ensue from removal of tonsils and adenoids. The improvement may, however, be due to removal of the chronic infective focus or to the correction of anoxia (associated with sleep apnoea – a significant and often unrecognised cause of poor growth). Children with severe intellectual deficit frequently grow poorly, sometimes as the result of feeding difficulties.

If, however, food intake is theoretically sufficient, and this can be convincingly documented (and in anorexic conditions this may not be easy), then presumably the food is being lost to the body, or is subject to an increased rate of metabolism. Some pathological states, for example, metabolic conditions, malignancies, and chronic infections, may cause weight loss and secondary poor growth through several possible mechanisms such as reduced appetite, vomiting, and other increased losses, and increased metabolism.

An adequate history and examination will often provide the diagnostic clues, but must clearly be aided by an awareness of possibilities.

Abnormal appearance

Many of the causes of children looking abnormal are underlying conditions which are associated with poor growth, or occasionally excessive growth. Some syndromes with growth implications are given on pp. 35–36, and discussed briefly in Chapter 10. Many of these are associated with poor growth in utero – born small for the length of gestation (so-called intrauterine growth retardation – see pp. 28–31).

Abnormal body proportions

Another feature of occasional diagnostic value is that of abnormal body proportions (see Box B). These may be very obvious, as in extreme forms of achondroplasia or Marfan's syndrome, but may not necessarily be so, and these cases can often be picked up by the simple procedures described in Chapter 2. Chronic lack of use of limbs results in their

> **Box B: Conditions with body disproportion**
>
> Short stature conditions with proportionately short limbs
>
> - Short limbed bone dysplasias, for example, achondroplasia, hypochondroplasia
> - Longstanding acquired hypothyroidism
> - Following extreme precocious puberty
>
> Short stature conditions with proportionately short trunk
>
> - Bone dysplasias primarily involving the spine
> - Severe spinal deformities – scoliosis, kyphosis
> - Following irradiation of the spine
>
> Tall stature conditions with proportionately long limbs
> - Marfan's syndrome
> - Klinefelter's syndrome
> - Following very delayed puberty (notably eunuchoidism)

poor growth, and this is found in severely paralysed limbs, notably in children with paraplegia, cerebral palsy, or severe arthritic conditions. The cause of poor growth here is usually obvious, though it is often not documented because of the technical difficulty of measurement. High dose irradiation markedly impairs the growth of bones within the irradiated field by a direct effect. A striking example of this is the shortening of the spine following spinal irradiation, for example, for pelvic, abdominal, thoracic, or spinal tumours, or leukaemia.

Puberty

The recognition of what is happening in terms of sexual development is fundamental to the evaluation of growth at an age when this may be relevant, as was considered in Chapter 6. At whatever age puberty or sexual development occurs, the sequence of accelerated growth followed by its deceleration and cessation is inevitable. The fact that the actual age at which this occurs is so variable within the overall population, means that it is impossible to evaluate the significance of height and weight at these ages without knowing the pubertal status.

70

Chronic ill health

The mechanisms whereby chronic illness results in poor growth are complex and multifactorial. Poor growth is the consequence of most long term conditions and may be due to the factors described as causing underweight (see Box A), but may also be the consequence of treatment (notably high dose steroids) and endocrine suppression, which may be psychologically dependent.

Psychosocial (emotional) deprivation

The adverse effects of severe psychosocial deprivation, as well as frank physical neglect and abuse, are well documented and undeniable. The situation is often associated with underfeeding, but the cause of the poor growth is more complex than this, for it occurs even when food intake is adequate and the child may be frankly obese. The lack of emotional input, with its severe psychological consequences, is one of the most powerful suppressors of growth. Sometimes there is secondary inhibition of endocrine function, notably growth hormone release, which is rapidly reversible if the cause can be recognised and corrected, yet treatment with the deficient hormone alone by no means guarantees a satisfactory growth response if the adverse circumstances persist.

It is often extremely difficult to recognise a psychosocial cause for poor growth, and even more difficult to prove and correct it, but it is most important to be aware of the possibility. Severe situations of this kind are unequivocally a cause of stunting of growth, but it is highly probable, though even harder to prove, that lesser degrees of emotional trauma, neglect, or psychological upset also take their toll in terms of reducing growth velocity, and it may be that quantitatively this is one of the commonest causes of growth retardation.

Failure to thrive

This term is used when a child fails to grow properly, but usually refers to a failure to gain weight in a child under the age of 2 – though it is also applicable to the developmental state. Although a minority of such children have an underlying medical problem, the cause is usually the consequence of undernutrition either through lack of food, because of poverty or neglect, or from problems with feeding. It is frequently indicative of difficulties in the mother–child relationship and other psychosocial problems in the family, being associated with poor psycho-motor development, emotional, and behavioural difficulties. As indicated above, physically or emotionally abused children often fail to thrive.

The normal expected weight and length gains in the first five years of life are indicated in Table 7.2; weights and lengths plotted on centile

Table 7.2   *Average gains in weight and length in the first five years of life*

Age	Increase in weight	Increase in length
0–1 week	Commonly lose up to 10% weight	
1 week–2 weeks	Birth weight regained	
2 weeks–5 months	150–200 g/week	
$4\frac{1}{2}$ months–5 months	Birth weight doubled	$1\cdot3 \times$ birth length
5 months–1 year	Weight gain progressively declines	
1 year	Birth weight almost trebled	$1\cdot5 \times$ birth length
1 year–2 years	2–3 kg in the year	11–12 cm in the year
2 years–5 years	Averaging 2 kg/year	Birth length doubled at about age 4

The increments are similar in boys and girls. The growth rate in first 1–2 years varies to take up the genetic potential, with either "catch up" in a baby small for dates or "catch down" in a large baby with a small father. The values in this table refer to babies born at term, and corrections must be applied for prematurity. Although the average baby may lose up to 10% body weight during the first week, some big babies lose more, and some "light for dates" babies may lose none at all.

charts should be corrected for prematurity (and this correction should be continued until the age of 2, when length measurements are usually changed to height with the consequent loss of about 1 cm).

In order to detect failure to thrive, measurements must be made regularly, but the frequency must represent a compromise between that necessary to recognise poor growth, and that which would cause needless worry (to the attendant as well as the parents) which can in itself be damaging. Weights may vary by several hundred grams depending on how full are the stomach, bowels, and bladder. The recommended measurements of infants (see Table 2.2 (p. 16)) will need to be more frequent if there are grounds for concern, and should then include length, head circumference, and mid-upper arm circumference, in addition to weight (see Table 2.5 (p. 27)). All clinic and surgery visits, whether for well baby checks or for illness, should include regular and recorded measurements.

Box C: Criteria for *initial* concern in infants less than 2 years old

Observations should be over sufficiently long intervals (more than one month), and not readily explicable, for example, by acute illness, and must be interpreted in the light of notes to Table 7.2

- Actual loss of weight
- Plateauing of weight to cross a major weight centile
- Weight repeatedly fluctuating up or down
- Weight below third centile
- Weight lying more than two major centiles below height

Suggested criteria for initial concern in infants under 2 years are listed in Box C, and would indicate the need for follow up every one to two months (the frequency depending on age). If the features causing concern persist, fuller evaluation by the primary care doctor (clinical medical officer or general practitioner) would be necessary to determine whether the growth is following a normal pattern or the concern is justified. This involves:

- Detailed history, particularly with regard to feeding, and the family growth pattern to obtain a mid-parental height centile;
- Clinical examination to note particularly: accurate length (without which correct interpretation of weight is impossible); head circumference; signs of wasting (mid-upper arm circumference, see Table 2.5); skinfolds; pallor; signs of neglect and maltreatment; developmental assessment;
- Consideration of health visitor's report on a home visit. This is a most helpful way of evaluating factors correlating to a child's growth, particularly if the baby or child can be observed at a meal time. Relevant aspects of such a visit are shown in Box D. Failure to thrive is diagnosed on the basis of growth data in conjunction with evidence of psychosocial problems and difficulties. In the majority of cases there is not an organic basis (although even in the minority when there is, a component of non-organic failure to thrive may be contributing to the poor growth). Organic causes can usually be excluded by clinical evaluation alone, allowing all concerned to focus appropriately on the real problem, and thus avoiding the multiple

73

Box D: Suggested areas for assessment by a health visitor at home

In the home	Is there evidence of financial, housing, or social difficulties (cold, damp, overcrowding)?
The family	Who are the principal caretakers?
	Are there problems of health, parenting abilities, or attitudes?
	Who else is part of the household?
	How is the family organised?
	Do other children have problems of health, growth, development, or behaviour?
The child	How is the child seen within the family?
	Is there concern shown about the child's weight gain, growth, development, health, behaviour, or temperament?
	Is psychomotor development appropriate for age?
Food	Is the child breast or bottle fed?
	Is the diet offered adequate in terms of quantity, quality, and frequency and timing of meals?
	How is the food prepared and served?
	Does the child have particular preferences and dislikes?
Feeding behaviour (by observation and discussion)	Are there feeding difficulties?
	How is the child positioned?
	Are there multiple and inconsistent feeders?
	Are there distractions or frequent interruptions?
	Are the meal times enjoyable?
	How much does the infant vomit or regurgitate?
	Is there open conflict between other family members during meals?
	Is there active withholding of food?

investigations or trials of different milk products which are expensive and obscure the real issues.

Management of children who are failing to thrive is considered in Chapter 9, referral to a consultant being appropriate with severe cases or when there are ongoing concerns that have not resolved with support from the health visitor and primary care doctor.

8: Laboratory diagnostic aids

It is not appropriate to discuss investigations in depth here, particularly those requiring admission of a child to hospital, so only brief consideration will be given, appropriate to community or outpatient settings.

The indications for investigations and the lines along which they should be directed will depend on the outcome of clinical evaluation and follow up, as described in the preceding chapters, and in Box A.

Investigations are only appropriate and justified following full clinical assessment, usually over a period of time, that has given sufficiently strong grounds for considering organic disease.

Routine investigations other than basic haematology and screening for urinary tract infection are not indicated. Bone age estimation, as indicated in Chapter 5, is a valuable diagnostic and predictive aid in many growth problems. Proposed basic outpatient investigations that can be considered for various conditions are outlined as below (normal values are shown in Appendix 3).

Outpatient investigations

Underweight with short stature

This category includes suspected organic failure to thrive.

Investigations should be directed to the effects of undernutrition and evidence of malabsorption or covert systemic disease.

Haematological studies

These comprise full blood count and film, erythrocyte sedimentation rate, or plasma viscosity. If the child proves anaemic, fuller haematological investigations to identify the type and cause of the anaemia may be indicated, for example, plasma ferritin, folate, reticulocytes, evidence of haemolysis, haemoglobin electrophoresis.

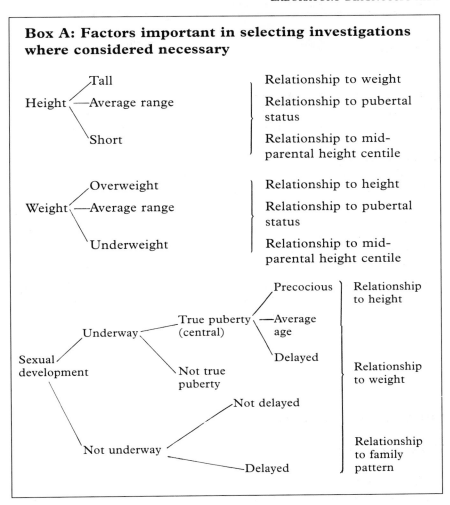

Box A: Factors important in selecting investigations where considered necessary

Other investigations

If symptoms and signs suggest malabsorption, in addition to the above the following investigations may be performed:

Stools	for ova and parasites;
Antibodies	for coeliac disease;
Sweat test	(and chest radiograph if there are respiratory symptoms) for cystic fibrosis.

Subsequent fuller investigations would require hospital attendance to diagnose coeliac disease (jejunal biopsy), chronic inflammatory bowel disease (radiological studies of the bowel), or specific studies to identify food intolerances.

Short stature and overweight

This combination, which is discussed in Chapter 4, raises the possibility of endocrine problems. It is only possible to undertake a few appropriate investigations on an outpatient basis, and these are outlined below.

Thyroid function tests

These are carried out to detect hypothyroidism (particularly if poor growth is associated with psychomotor delay).

Screening growth hormone tests

In normal healthy individuals, growth hormone levels in the blood are low for most of the time, with only occasional short lasting spikes, either spontaneous or in response to physiological effects – notably severe exercise, and sleep. Random sampling, which by chance is likely to yield a low growth hormone level, is seldom helpful as a means of excluding deficiency. (In contrast, it will usually be satisfactory in excluding overproduction when the rare circumstance of excessive growth hormone production is suspected.) Box B outlines the ways in which growth hormone status can be investigated in practice.

Other investigations into endocrine function

Other investigations, such as fuller growth hormone studies, investigation of possible overproduction of glucocorticoids or evaluation of diabetic control in poorly growing patients with diabetes, would require hospital admission.

Short stature not specifically linked with over- or underweight

This possibility exists without the usual weight associations described, and testing for it may be appropriate if other evidence is sufficiently suggestive. There are, however, a few other simpler outpatient procedures which may be considered in the appropriate circumstances, usually of a screening nature.

Box B: Plasma or serum growth hormone levels in diagnosis

To exclude deficiency – in short stature conditions
The demonstration of a high level is required
Random levels are usually low
Specific stimuli are usually necessary:

Physiological screening procedures

- Intensive exercise (single blood sample taken 25 minutes after the start of 10 minutes intensive exercise)
- Sleep (usually impractical as a screening test, as it requires sampling around the time of onset of deep sleep)

Pharmacological screening procedure

- Requires hospitalisation with serial half-hourly blood sampling over $2\frac{1}{2}$–3 hours following an appropriate stimulus of which there are many – the commonest in use nowadays are intramuscular glucagon, intravenous arginine infusion, and oral clonidine. Intravenous insulin to induce hypoglycaemia used to be the gold standard, but is seldom used now because of the occasional occurrence of severe or even fatal complications

To exclude overproduction – in tall stature conditions
The demonstration of a low level is required.
A random level (if necessary repeated) is usually sufficient. If this is persistently high, suppression by high blood glucose levels (through a glucose tolerance test with repeated sampling over $2\frac{1}{2}$–3 hours) is needed, requiring attendance at hospital

[Urinary growth hormone assays are available in a few centres and, though not widely used at present, may well become a convenient and acceptable alternative to blood testing if the method can be validated. This would merely involve collecting urine overnight.]

Basic biochemical profile and urinalysis

These tests are performed to identify or exclude renal insufficiency, urinary tract infections, hepatic disease, diabetes mellitus, diabetes insipidus, or other rarer metabolic conditions. Subsequent management and fuller investigation would be at a hospital level.

Chromosome analysis

This is essential for the diagnosis of Turner's syndrome, of which there should be a high level of suspicion in any girl with unexplained short stature, even in the absence of any of the other classical features of the condition. The investigation is also often indicated in dysmorphic conditions with a constellation of abnormal features, some of which are linked with an abnormal chromosomal constitution.

Radiological studies

Apart from bone age investigations and chest radiographs, these would seldom be appropriate on an outpatient basis.

Suspected bone dysplasias (short stature conditions frequently with body disproportion) are diagnosed on the basis of specific abnormalities on skeletal surveys. (These are also undertaken for totally different reasons to reveal fractures in suspected child abuse and non-accidental injury.)

Tuberculin testing

This is occasionally indicated, particularly with immigrant children, but chronic tuberculosis in childhood is rarely the cause of poor growth.

Tall stature and overweight

This seldom requires investigation as it is usually exogenous, not the result of organic disease. Bone age estimation indicating physiological advancement (which is self evident if puberty is under way) is reassuring in confirming this type of obesity.

Tall stature and underweight

In the majority of children of this type, a familial basis is the explanation, as it is with all types of tall stature in childhood, and only rarely is investigation needed. Rare conditions are juvenile hyperthyroidism, for which thyroid function tests would be the proof, and Marfan's syndrome, to be discussed later (Chapter 10), for which in the absence of pathognomonic eye signs there are no specific diagnostic investigations. The metacarpal index, which is the ratio of the length to the width of the largest metacarpal on a hand radiograph, is reputed to be greater than 8·4 in this condition, but a diagnosis founded on that measurement would be very dubious.

Extreme tall stature not specifically linked with over- or underweight

Tall stature is rarely due to an underlying pathology and the common explanations of tall parents, advanced physiological age and puberty (and exogenous obesity) do not require investigation. In the rare circumstance when tallness cannot be accounted for in this way, investigations may be indicated.

Chromosome analysis

This will identify the trisomies 47,XXY (Klinefelter's syndrome) and 47,XYY, which are difficult to diagnose clinically (see Chapter 10).

Hormone analyses

As already indicated, these tests are necessary to diagnose the very rare conditions of excessive production causing tall stature in childhood – hyperthyroidism or pituitary gigantism. Random thyroid function levels will confirm or refute the former diagnosis, and, as indicated in Box B, a low random growth hormone level usually excludes growth hormone excess as the cause. The investigation of the tallness associated with precocious sexual development is considered separately.

Precocious sexual development

This condition, as the cause of excessive tallness at the time (although ultimately causing short stature), has been considered in Chapter 6. Investigations when necessary are directed more at identifying the cause, and careful clinical examination is usually sufficient to show that sexual development is under way.

Bone age

Bone age estimation is valuable to indicate the degree of physiological advancement and reduction of growth potential.

Hormone analyses

Plasma levels of oestrogens, androgens, and gonadotrophins (luteinising hormone and follicle stimulating hormone) are seldom helpful, merely confirming what is clinically obvious. However, in some situations where it is unclear whether the sexual development represents true central precocious puberty or not, these estimations may be of value. Sexual development in boys, dependent on hormones from a non-testicular source, or exclusively androgenic features in a developing girl, may be shown by low plasma gonadotrophins and higher levels of plasma adrenal androgens (androstenedione, dehydroepiandrosterone, 17α-hydroxyprogesterone – if markedly elevated, the last is almost diagnostic of congenital adrenal hyperplasia, which may present much later than the newborn period). Testosterone will be proportionately less elevated.

Other investigations

Further investigation and treatment of these rare conditions of ambiguity of sexual development and true precocious puberty require specialised investigation in hospital, including radiological investigations, ultrasound scanning of the pelvis and abdomen to outline and identify gonads and internal genitalia, and the adrenal glands, and computed tomography or magnetic resonance imaging of these areas and the brain.

Delayed sexual development

This will be associated with a fall off in height and weight centile position, but assuming sexual development does occur ultimately, the growth will continue to an older age and final adult height will be better in terms of centile position, or even frankly tall. As discussed in Chapter 6, the age at which the delay warrants investigation usually depends more on family concerns than on purely clinical grounds. The simple outpatient investigations described below would then be carried out.

Bone age

This would be assessed to indicate the degree of physiological delay and degree of residual growth.

Chromosome analysis

In primary gonadal failure, chromosome analysis is indicated in short stature girls to identify Turner's syndrome (45,XO karyotypes or mosaics or loss of a component of the second X) and in males to identify Klinefelter's syndrome (47,XXY). The testes are invariably very small but, though incapable of producing many viable sperm, may yet produce testosterone in variable amounts with consequent varying degrees of virilisation.

Hormone analyses

Levels of luteinising hormone and follicle stimulating hormone are measured to determine whether the cause of the delay is gonadal (when pituitary gonadotrophin output will be high) or hypothalamic–pituitary (when plasma gonadotrophins will be low, as this lack is the cause of the delay).

Hospital procedures are also required in secondary gonadal failure, where the presence of low plasma gonadotrophins may be due to a failure either of hypothalamic luteinising hormone releasing hormone (LHRH) production and release, or of pituitary gonadotrophin release, which may be of organic origin or simply due to physiological delay.

The value of the LHRH stimulation test in this situation is controversial, but involves sampling plasma half-hourly for 90 minutes following an intravenous bolus injection of LHRH. The pattern of gonadotrophin release is an indication of potential pituitary responsiveness, and may give a clue as to whether puberty is imminent and when.

Early morning (8.00 am) plasma testosterone estimation in boys showing a level over 0·9 mmol/l is a good indication that delay is physiological and features of puberty are likely to appear within a year.

The gonadotrophin stimulation test, by demonstrating the oestradiol response in girls or testosterone response in boys 48 hours after a large bolus of gonadotrophin, is an indication of potential gonadal hormone function, and in cryptorchid boys whether viable testicular tissue exists. In girls, investigation specifically of delayed menarche is only necessary if normal puberty has progressed satisfactorily; if not, then the relevant investigations are those indicated above for overall pubertal delay, for menarche itself is merely a late feature depending on preceding normal progress in puberty.

Other investigations

It is important to identify whether there are gonads in primary gonadal failure, and, if so, whether there is likely to be any potential function on the basis of their size. This may be achieved by ultrasound examination but may require laparoscopy, especially in cryptorchid boys; these are both hospital procedures.

9: Treatment of growth disorders

Basic considerations regarding appropriateness of treatment of growth disorders

Whether it is appropriate to institute treatment with regard to growth, and the form that treatment will take depend on many considerations,

---

Box A: Factors to consider in determining whether and how to treat growth disorders

Who is the person concerned?

What is the level of concern?

Why is there concern?

Is there an identifiable pathological cause?

Is there a specific treatment?

How beneficial and justifiable are non-specific treatments?

---

some of which are suggested in Box A. It is firstly relevant to know who or what initiated the concern (Chapter 2, Box B (p. 17)). This is by no means always the child or parents themselves, for their reaction to similar degrees of fatness or thinness, tallness or shortness varies considerably. The short children of short parents, or the tall children of tall parents may be quite content, and rightly so, to attribute their stature to inheritance, and whether or not the parents are concerned about the growth of their children may well depend on how bothered they themselves have been through childhood and as adults. Perhaps, sadly, this attitude may be coloured by that of society, and in particular the media which often suggest that success and happiness in life are related to tallness – particularly in men.

Children will inevitably compare their stature and physique with those of the people with whom they associate, particularly at school where comments are bound to be made by other pupils, teachers, and school nurses or doctors. The medical profession may become aware of a child's atypical growth as a result of the screening procedures described in Chapter 2, or because specific problems, either directly or indirectly related to growth, have led to attendance at the clinic or surgery. It is important that concern engendered in the child or parents is appropriate, for in some situations it is of the utmost importance that abnormal growth is recognised and treated early, whereas in others intervention may not be beneficial or may even be detrimental by creating unnecessary anxiety and concern.

The grounds on which individuals base their concern will also vary, as considered in Chapter 2, Box C (p. 17). These may be justified or not, notably depending on whether or not there is an underlying pathology linked to the growth picture. Such a pathology may be progressive and cause other significant or serious features in addition to those related to growth. In such circumstances appropriate treatment, if it is available, is nearly always indicated. In the absence of such a diagnosis, treatment must be less specific and its appropriateness and form are much less well defined and may be controversial. Though short term benefit is often valuable, it is the long term outcome that is usually the major consideration, and if this is not likely to be improved sufficiently as the result of treatment then its use may well be in question. In some situations, notably in regard to the atypical timing of puberty, the ultimate outcome may be satisfactory without treatment, and that knowledge may in itself provide sufficient reassurance.

General review of treatment

Treatment can thus be considered from many aspects. Some medical treatments are unequivocally appropriate for specific conditions as indicated in Box B and discussed further below. Other medical treatments are, however, less well defined and not necessarily universally agreed and some of these are listed in Box C.2 and will also be considered later. However, to achieve the best response to a specific medical treatment involves much more than just the medicines, namely other treatment modalities and the involvement of many different individuals. Complete care of the child – and family – involves many facets, as suggested in Box C.1.

Optimal growth requires adequate nutrition and a stable environment free from excessive psychological, emotional, and physical stress, with

Box B: Specific treatments for specific pathologies causing abnormal growth

1 *Hormonal abnormalities*	*Treatment*
Hormone deficiency, for example: • Thyroid deficiency • Growth hormone deficiency • Deficiency of gonadal hormones or gonadotrophins	Appropriate replacement
Hormone excess, for example: • Hyperthyroidism • Growth hormone excess • Glucocorticoid excess • Sex hormone excess	Suppression or removal of the cause

2 *Nutritional abnormalities*

Undernutrition • Inadequate intake in quantity or quality	Provision of appropriate foods
• Malabsorptions: Coeliac disease Fibrocystic disease Food allergies and intolerances Inflammatory bowel disease	Directed to the primary pathology
• Chronic diseases	Optimal appropriate treatment
• Psychological disturbance or emotional upset	Appropriate psychological and social support, or change of environment and caring programme, or both
Overnutrition • Obesity	Appropriate dieting and exercise (plus specific treatment if there is an underlying cause)

Box C: Non-specific treatments for growth disorders

1 General supportive measures
- Improved general health – Treatment of chronic disease
                           – Appropriate and adequate food intake
                           – Exercise

- Psychological evaluation, support, and counselling

- Aids to living, notably in the home, for those with short stature

- Improvement of the environment – notably in circumstances of psychosocial deprivation and psychological stress

2 Medical treatments in situations without specific indications (Mostly controversial to some degree)

Hormones

- to promote or accelerate growth, for example, growth hormone, sex hormones, gonadotrophins, anabolic steroids

- to suppress or delay growth and sexual development

- to speed on and terminate puberty, such as in tall stature

Diets, such as:

- exclusion diets in suspected food intolerances or sensitivities

- addition of specific components, for example, vitamins, iron, calcium, trace minerals

Surgical procedures, such as:

- limb lengthening

- correction of spinal deformities

---

the positive aspects of stimulation, affection, and encouragement. To achieve this requires a team to share the care which, though often centred upon the hospital paediatrician, is more a partnership in which each member's role is important and complementary (see Box D).

Box D: Staff involved in various aspects of treatment – shared care

Doctors

- Hospital paediatric consultant, and clinical assistants
- General practitioner
- Community paediatrician and community doctors (school doctors)

In particular circumstances:

- Other specialists, such as surgeons, psychiatrists, gynaecologists

Nurses

- in clinic
- in community, health visitors, outreach nurses, et cetera

Psychologists

Dietitians

Parents and family (or other carers)

Others for specific aspects, such as radiologists, pharmacists, laboratory staff, physiotherapists, social workers, et cetera

---

Medical personnel

Depending on the nature of the problem, the *doctor* most involved on an ongoing basis may be the general practitioner, the local community or hospital paediatrician, or a paediatric endocrinologist or growth specialist. Some degree of shared care is usually possible and preferable with ready means of communication. The frequency of attendance with the specialist or local paediatrician, and where this will be, will vary depending on the complexity of the disease and its management, as well as on the ease and distance of travel, et cetera. Combined clinics at district hospitals involving specialists and local doctors are valuable, as are those between adult orientated specialists and the paediatrician, particularly in the care of those children who are passing through adolescence and are likely to require continuing care as adults.

Nurse input is invaluable. In the clinic situation the experienced nurse, in addition to more obvious practical nursing duties, has a unique opportunity through observation and conversation with the children and their families to bring to light and clarify problems and difficulties of many kinds which have a bearing on the child's well being, progress, and response to treatment. The doctor in the clinic may not be aware of these aspects, because of pressure of time or the disinclination or reticence of the family members to proffer these concerns to a doctor. However, out of the clinic setting, before or after seeing the doctor, patients and their families are often more forthcoming and less inhibited and will talk to a familiar friendly nurse who has the insight to give them the opportunity to do so.

In the home, too, nurses have a crucial role. They may provide an outreach service from the hospital and often be already known through the clinic, or may be community nurses or health visitors, sometimes linked with a general practice. Their input has many facets. They can give instruction in treatment procedures (such as injection techniques), supervise these, and check that they are undertaken correctly, and get some idea of compliance. They can clarify aspects that are not fully understood, relieve anxieties, and answer a host of questions. Being in the home they have a unique opportunity to see at first hand the environment in which the child is being brought up, to recognise adverse effects of poverty, overcrowding, friction, or neglect, or, conversely, be able to provide reassurance that all is well. By being made aware of these elements, the doctor is in a much better position to evaluate the effect of treatment and to recognise factors that may have contributed to a poor response, and to attempt, at least in theory, to rectify them.

Psychological support should be available to the hospital clinic, but how much it is required or used varies greatly and depends on the attitude of the medical staff, their insight into problems, and the resources at their disposal. There is no doubt that there is a critical interplay between the psychological and physical condition of children, par- ticularly those with growth problems.[15] Psychological problems may be very marked and obvious, but they may also be hidden and subtle and yet of great relevance. Children who are at extremes of short or tall stature, fatness or thinness, or advanced or retarded in puberty are exposed to great emotional and physical stresses, which may in them- selves have an adverse effect on growth and response to treatment. In addition, adverse psychological factors are themselves sometimes the underlying cause of poor growth. Every effort should be made to provide the means of identifying these problems and to have trained staff to help overcome them. Counselling involves all the members of the family, but success in every aspect of management, whether or not there are emotional and psychological problems, can only be fully achieved by having the support, understanding, and sympathy of those caring for the child in the home. Sadly, that is frequently not possible, but it should certainly be the goal.

The involvement of the *dietitian* is an essential component in the management of many children with growth problems. These aspects are basically obvious and are shown in Box E. The input of the dietitian is

---

Box E: The role of the dietitian

Evaluation of the composition of the current diet in:	*Advice on dietary adjustment and how to achieve it*
Suspected general undernutrition (and cystic fibrosis)	General increase in protein or calorie intake, or both
Suspected specific deficiencies, for example, iron, vitamins, calcium, et cetera	Appropriate supplementation
Obesity	Supervised reduction in food intake
Suspected food intolerances	Elimination diets in specific conditions, for example:
	Food intolerance, for example, to cow's milk protein, egg, soya, food additives, (NB dangers of unnecessary dietary restrictions in some types of "allergic" diseases)
	Coeliac disease: gluten avoidance (and sometimes transiently disaccharides)

---

frequently ongoing, and the aspects often need regular review particularly when response to treatment is disappointing. Liaison with other members of the "team", often within the clinic setting, is important, both for exchange of information and for evaluating compliance. Dietitians provide advice relating to exclusion diets, by identifying unnecessary dietary restrictions, and assessing the adequacy of diets that may have been undertaken misguidedly. They also advise on reintroduction of foods that had been withdrawn with little clinical justification in an attempt to prove intolerance.

Surgical procedures

In addition to the surgery required in particular clinical conditions – for example, tumours, orthopaedic problems et cetera – limb lengthening procedures are occasionally undertaken in children with extreme short stature. This is a developing field where the indications at present are limited but may increase in the future. Such surgery is undertaken in only a few centres and usually involves a prolonged period of immobility; however, the increase in stature achieved is considerable, and rapid compared with other treatments. It is most appropriate in disproportionate short limbed conditions, notably achondroplasia; here the procedure corrects the disproportion and, as the tissues overlying the short bones are frequently redundant, lengthening the bones takes up this slack, in contrast to other short stature conditions where such tissues would be put under abnormal tension.

General principles regarding treatment

1 In any acquired (as distinct from congenital) growth problem due to hormonal dysfunction, an underlying cause should be sought, which should if possible be treated in its own right.
2 The best and most effective treatments are those specific for the condition, for example:
   ● hormone deficiency – replacing with that particular hormone
   ● excluding a specific dietary factor responsible for the disease.
3 Growth response to appropriate specific medication will not be fully effective if:
   ● there is inadequate nutrition

- there is a psychological or emotional upset
- there is an ongoing active chronic disease process
- there is poor compliance.

4 There is no value in any treatment to promote growth when there is no residual growth potential, that is, when the epiphyses have fused at the end of puberty.

5 Growth is still possible in response to appropriate treatment as long as puberty is not completed – whatever the actual age.

6 Hormone replacements should mimic the normal physiological pattern of release as much as realistically possible.

7 In treating multiple hormone deficiencies, correct dosage of *all* deficient hormones is necessary for optimal response.

8 Inappropriately high dosage and prolonged treatment with many hormones (for example, glucocorticoids, oestrogens, androgens, gonadotrophins, anabolic agents) may result in *ultimate* height being stunted as well as causing other side effects.

9 A child deficient in growth promoting hormones, but who is in puberty, may erroneously be assumed to be growing satisfactorily, whereas in fact the growth velocity is less than it should be and growth prognosis will be poor without full hormone replacement.

Treatment with drugs

A brief outline of drug treatment of growth disorders is given in Table 9.1. The detailed management and adjustment of dosage is usually best undertaken in a hospital clinic. Many alternative preparations are available, but only one commonly used preparation is cited as an example in each group.

Growth hormone treatment

Only two indications, growth hormone deficiency and Turner's syndrome, have official approval. Children with unequivocal growth hormone deficiency should respond well to growth hormone treatment, but the response to treatment of those with so-called "partial" deficiencies (with growth hormone levels on pharmacological testing between 10 and 20 U/l) is less predictable. Many of the latter may be wrongly diagnosed as such, particularly in situations of delayed puberty, and prove to grow satisfactorily without treatment when puberty occurs.

Drug	Indications	Dosage	Route	Duration	Comments
Carbimazole	Hyperthyroidism	15–30 mg daily divided into three 8 hourly doses	Oral	Variable (usually about 2 years)	Dose gradually reduced and adjusted according to clinical condition and blood levels of T_4 and TSH (concomitant thyroxine 50 μg daily advisable)
Desmopressin (DDAVP)	Diabetes insipidus	5–20 μg daily usually divided into two doses	Intranasal	Lifelong	Dose adjusted according to clinical state
Ethinyloestradiol (oestrogen)	Female hypogonadism, primary or secondary	Gradual increase over several years from 1 μg daily to adult dose of ≥ 20 μg	Oral	Lifelong	Initial dose must be very low and the increase gradual to avoid premature epiphyseal fusion
Fludrocortisone (mineralocorticoid)	Physiological replacement in adrenal insufficiency	50–200 μg daily divided into two doses (5 μg/kg)	Oral	Lifelong	Dose adjusted in relation to plasma electrolytes and renin activity (if available) and to avoid hypertension
Growth hormone (see text)	1 Growth hormone deficiency	0·6 U/kg/week divided into daily doses	Subcutaneous injection	(a) until an acceptable height is achieved or (b) until growth is almost complete, but (c) only if a reasonable height velocity is maintained	
	2 Turner's syndrome	1·0 U/kg/week divided into daily doses	Subcutaneous injection	As above. Response better in younger children and falls off in the teens	
Hydrocortisone (glucocorticoids – see text)	Physiological replacement in adrenal insufficiency	20 mg/m² divided into two doses: $\frac{2}{3}$ in morning, $\frac{1}{3}$ in evening, or three doses	Oral	Lifelong	Dose tailored to needs and to avoid adverse effects on growth (and to biochemistry in congenital adrenal hyperplasia). Dose increased at times of stress
Sustanon (androgen)	1 Male hypogonadism primary or secondary	Gradual increase from 50 mg monthly to adult dose of 250 mg every 3 weeks	Intramuscular injection	Lifelong	
	2 To trigger puberty	50–100 mg monthly	Intramuscular injection	3–6 months	
Thyroxine (T_4)	Hypothyroidism	3–5 μg/kg daily	Oral	Lifelong	Dose adjusted according to clinical condition and blood levels of T_4 and TSH

Growth hormone has been used in high dosage in many other short stature conditions, but such treatment is controversial and probably not justified at present except as part of well monitored clinical trials. True growth hormone deficiency may be associated with deficiencies of other anterior pituitary trophic hormones (and occasionally also diabetes insipidus) and incorrect replacement dosage of these hormones, for example, thyroid hormones, or excessive glucocorticoid replacement, may result in a suboptimal growth response.

Biosynthetic growth hormone preparations are produced by several pharmaceutical companies and the efficacy and cost of these are similar. There are, however, different formulations and multidose vials and "pen devices" are popular, convenient, and simple to use after instruction. Human growth hormone derived from human pituitary glands was withdrawn totally in 1985, following its identification as the cause of the few cases of the fatal condition Creutzfeldt–Jakob disease.

Glucocorticoid treatment

In relation to growth disorders glucocorticoids are used as replacement for deficiency in physiological dosage which, if correctly determined, should not be growth suppressant. When used in other conditions, for example, asthma, juvenile chronic arthritis, malignancies, nephrotic syndrome, et cetera, doses are much larger and pharmacological. These higher doses do suppress growth, though the precise levels required to do so vary from individual to individual and depend also on the condition being treated. As a guideline in these conditions, doses equivalent to less than 50 mg per square metre surface area per day of cortisone or hydrocortisone are not growth suppressant. Yet in treatment of panhypopituitarism and some other causes of adrenal insufficiency, much lower dosage of glucocorticoids may have an inhibitory effect on growth and the appropriate dose requires careful adjustment. (Prednisone and prednisolone are 10 times more potent in their growth suppressant effects than cortisone.) As already indicated, high dosage of inhaled steroids and steroids absorbed through the skin can also cause growth suppression.

Tall stature

As indicated previously (pp. 31–36) tall stature is seldom pathological but is sometimes embarrassing and inconvenient. It is important before contemplating treatment directed to lessening potential adult height to have predicted what that height is likely to be and that it would be unacceptable. As with short stature, what seems unacceptable varies greatly from individual to individual, and is more often a concern with girls than boys. As a common cause of tall stature in the growing years is "physiological advancement and puberty at an earlier than average age", prediction will then often show that ultimate stature will not be excessive.[14] In general, adult heights of less than 183 cm (6'0") for girls and considerably taller for boys would not justify treatment. When treatment is considered, this should not be undertaken lightly but following full discussion, as benefit cannot be guaranteed nor can the possibility of long term sequelae be ignored. However, an essential consideration if treatment is contemplated is that it must not be left until too late, to a time when the child has already reached a stature close to that which would be unacceptable for the adult.

The principle underlying what used to be the commonest form of treatment was to accelerate fusion of the epiphyses by speeding up the pubertal process with very high doses of oestrogen in girls (of the order of 300 µg ethinyloestradiol daily) or testosterone in boys (for example, Sustanon 500 mg fortnightly). There is, however, considerable doubt whether this treatment is effective, and even if it is, whether it is any more so than using sex hormones in much lower dosage. The treatment should not be instituted at an age so young that it would be unacceptable for the child to be in puberty, or in girls to menstruate, yet not left so late that there is insufficient time remaining to achieve any significant benefit. Treatment would be continued until epiphyses had fused or the prediction for adult height had lessened to an acceptable degree.

An alternative treatment which could be initiated at a much younger age, as it is not dependent on inducing or speeding up puberty, is to reduce growth hormone release using somatostatin analogues (for example, octreotide). Unfortunately, these drugs are not yet available for general use in the United Kingdom, though they have proved beneficial in trials in specialist centres. In the future, when predictions indicate a poor outcome without treatment, the approach will probably be to start treatment at a prepubertal age with somatostatin and continue this until the earliest age at which puberty could be acceptably induced.

Precocious sexual development

The treatment of this condition depends on the underlying cause.

If sexual precocity is not dependent on central gonadotrophin drive, the underlying cause of the excessive production of sex hormones will need treating, for example, by removal of an adrenal tumour or the replacement of deficient glucocorticoids and mineralocorticoids in late presenting congenital adrenal hyperplasia.

If the puberty is "central", that is, gonadotrophin dependent, the following considerations are appropriate:

1 If there is an underlying pathology, such as intracranial tumour, this should be treated in its own right if possible.
2 Treatment to delay puberty is indicated, firstly
  (a) if the age is so young as to be socially and psychologically unacceptable, and
  (b) if predicted adult height would be unacceptably short because of premature epiphyseal fusion.

Treatment is continued until an age is reached when pubertal changes would be acceptable or when there is the likelihood of a satisfactory adult height being achieved.

The most effective treatments nowadays are the gonadotrophin releasing hormone analogues. By maintaining a continual high level these effectively switch off gonadotrophin release, but they have the disadvantage that compliance with treatment is essential, otherwise an opposite effect to that desired will result. The intranasal forms of treatment (buserelin or nafarelin) have largely been superseded by longacting preparations administered monthly by injection (goserelin or leuprorelin). These treatments are effective both in stopping progress or reversing pubertal features and in improving height prognosis. Other treatments which are easier to administer are less effective with regard to height. These act by antigonadotrophin progestogenic properties: cyproterone acetate orally, $60–100 \, mg/m^2/day$ in three divided doses, or alternatively girls may receive medroxyprogesterone acetate (Provera) 100 mg every two weeks by intramuscular injection.

Delayed puberty

The implications of this have already been considered (see pp. 64–65). If the delay is due to an underlying pathology either at a gonadal or hypothalamic–pituitary level, then long term gonadal hormone replacement will be necessary. This would be started at an age comparable to the normal population but in a very low dose, gradually building up over three to four years to the adult levels. Much more commonly the delay is physiological, and treatment for three to six months only, to trigger off puberty should be sufficient, and on stopping this puberty will usually subsequently progress spontaneously. The indications for this treatment will be based on the age and height centile of the child, and the degree of stress and emotional upset engendered. In boys the most common treatment advocated is testosterone (Sustanon 100 mg monthly by intramuscular injection). An alternative is human chorionic gonadotrophin which, though theoretically more physiological, is less acceptable because it requires more frequent intramuscular injections (1000 international units twice weekly). Treatment for delayed puberty is far less commonly required in girls than boys, but when it is, is probably best achieved with low dose oestrogen. Oxandrolone, a weakly anabolic agent (taken orally in a dose of 1·25–2·5 mg daily for three to six months) is another possible treatment (in either sex), but can only be prescribed on a named patient basis from hospital. This is reported to accelerate growth, but the effect is unpredictable; it is usually, but not invariably linked with the induction of puberty, although a response is more likely if puberty is imminent. It remains to be seen whether ultimate height would be jeopardised by inappropriate advancement of bone age.

10: Examples of growth disorders

This chapter first describes common growth problems, and outlines briefly the salient clinical features of the conditions. In the second part there are 35 case histories illustrating these conditions.

Conditions with short stature

Familial (non-pathological)

As shown in Chapter 3, Box D, the expected influence of inheritance on the height of a child can be indicated by the mid-parental centile, and is by far the commonest explanation for short (or tall) stature in childhood, although when there is a marked difference between the height centiles of the mother and father, the child may have taken after either. The timing of puberty may also show some inherited pattern linked with "physiological" advancement or retardation, but evidenced before puberty only by the skeletal age. Of course, many features other than stature, such as body build, et cetera, will normally be inherited (see case 21).

Undernutrition

If this is the cause of short stature, weight is usually more affected (that is, at a lower centile) than height. The slowing down in height velocity follows that of weight and may take several months before its effect is evident, whereas marked weight changes can occur rapidly. That poor weight represents undernutrition can be confirmed by low skinfold and mid-upper arm circumference measurements.

Inadequate intake of food

This may be due to failure to offer sufficient or appropriate food, either through ignorance, poverty, or neglect, or to the many causes of poor appetite (see Chapter 3). A detailed, reliable assessment of dietary intake is very helpful in relation to this diagnosis.

Examples:

Psychosocial and emotional causes of poor growth may involve inadequate food intake, but this is not the whole explanation (see Chapter 3). There is commonly delay in development. The severity of the underlying psychological "trauma" may range from overt abuse and neglect to much more subtle causes, difficult to identify and even more difficult to prove. (See Case 1.)

Poor food intake due to upper airway obstruction and chronic upper respiratory infections. (See Case 2.)

Anorexia nervosa: most commonly occurring in the pubertal age range, children (girls eight times more frequently than boys) become obsessed with losing weight, mistakenly considering themselves overweight. They claim to be fit and energetic, and the dieting may be secretive and associated with induced vomiting. Pubertal changes cease or regress, the menarche is delayed or menstrual periods stop. (See Case 3.)

Malabsorption

This diagnosis can be suspected on the basis of chronically abnormal bowel symptoms (though these are not invariable), wasting, and protuberant abdomen. Additional features point to the specific diagnoses: recurrent respiratory infections, yet cheerful personality and reasonable appetite with cystic fibrosis; poor appetite and misery with coeliac disease, the features not developing until the infant is weaned. (See Case 4.)

Poor growth and undernutrition may also be due to chronic inflammatory bowel disease, for example, Crohn's disease.

Endocrine

Short stature is usually associated with weight that is at a better centile position than height, often with frank obesity and increased skinfold measurements.

Examples:

Acquired hypothyroidism: features usually develop insidiously, notably with poor growth, sluggish behaviour, constipation, lack of energy, and a bloated (myxoedematous) appearance. Presentation is sometimes due to the orthopaedic effects of epiphysial dysgenesis (notably in the hips). Intellectual impairment is seldom commented on (in marked contrast to the inevitable consequence of late diagnosed cretinism, or congenital hypothyroidism, which hopefully will seldom be seen nowadays because of neonatal screening), and children who when hypothyroid are docile may present more behavioural problems (perhaps normal ones!) when they become euthyroid with treatment. Confirmatory features are bradycardia, tendon reflexes which relax slowly after a normal contraction phase, and very retarded bone ages. The commonest cause in childhood is autoimmune thyroiditis (Hashimoto's disease) but a goitre is only occasionally found. (See Cases 5, 6 and 26.)

Growth hormone deficiency: whether or not this is congenital or acquired later in childhood, such children most commonly present because of poor growth (unless the diagnosis is anticipated because of known pathologies in the region of the hypothalamus and pituitary, and the degree of short stature will then depend on the interval from the onset of the pathology). Other features are the relative obesity, crowding of mid-facial structures and retardation of bone age. The condition is commoner in boys and those born by breech delivery. Deficiency may be isolated or multiple, involving other pituitary hormones when appropriate features will also be present, including sometimes polydipsia and polyuria due to diabetes insipidus, hypoglycaemia in infancy and micropenis. Diabetes insipidus, acquired after infancy, caused by antidiuretic hormone deficiency from the posterior pituitary, is commonly the result of progressive underlying pathology and warrants full investigation, as well as an awareness that it may be accompanied by deficiencies of anterior pituitary hormones. (See Cases 7, 8 and 9.)

Glucocorticoid excess is rarely due to pituitary or adrenal disease in childhood and is much more commonly the result of treatment with high dosage glucocorticoids. As well as short stature and obesity, which is most markedly truncal, there may be purple striae, a tendency to bruising, a plethoric moon face, hirsuties, hypertension, and muscle weakness. The dose of steroids necessary to produce growth retardation is not rigidly definable, varying considerably from individual to individual. A dose of oral steroid equivalent to 35 mg cortisone/m^2 is frequently growth suppressant, as are inhaled steroids for asthma, for example, doses of beclomethasone greater than 800 µg/day, but in some individuals lower doses may slow down growth rate. (See Cases 10 and 11.)

Delayed puberty whether physiological or pathological will result in

100

short stature but with the prospect of catch up ultimately when the pubertal growth has occurred (see Chapter 6 and Cases 22 and 23).

Bone dysplasias

The clue to this diagnostic group, if it is not clinically obvious as it is in achondroplasia, is body disproportion with atypical limb to trunk proportions. In short-limbed conditions the weight centile is usually at a higher level than the height centile, not necessarily due to obesity but because of the greater proportionate weight contribution from the upper body segment than from the legs. Many of these conditions are inherited. (See Cases 12, 13 and 14.)

Specific "syndromes" associated with short stature

The children have abnormal appearances with features indicating the diagnosis. They mostly show intrauterine growth retardation and inappropriately low birth weight, and grow poorly from the start.

Down's syndrome: the classical features are familiar and include characteristic facial appearance with upward sloping palpebral fissures and epicanthic folds, protruding tongue, small ears, flat occiput, single palmar creases and incurved little fingers, with a wide gap between the first and second toes. They usually have mild to moderate mental retardation. Congenital heart disease occurs in nearly half the cases. Height centile charts are available for Down's syndrome. (See Case 15.)

Turner's syndrome: the spectrum of possible features of this condition is very large, and the only almost invariable feature is short stature.

In the majority, however, there is a failure of puberty and menstruation (and infertility) due to ovarian dysgenesis. The lack of a full X chromosome of the classical condition occurs only in about two thirds of cases, and these are the ones more likely to show some of the other features, such as peripheral oedema in infancy, web neck (or short neck and low posterior hair line), increased carrying angle at the elbow (cubitus valgus), shield-shaped chest with widely spaced nipples, high arched palate, multiple small pigmented naevi, defective nails, recurrent otitis media and deafness, and congenital heart disease of which coarctation of the aorta (rare otherwise in girls) is the most common. The complete range of these characteristics is seldom seen.

The remaining third have a mosaic chromosome pattern, or a loss of only a part of an X chromosome, and some of these girls may look in no way abnormal apart from being short of stature.

Height centile charts for girls with Turner's syndrome are available and the mean ultimate height (untreated) is only about 143 cm (see Cases 16 and 17).

Noonan's syndrome: the features of this condition are superficially similar to those of Turner's syndrome, and it used to be termed "male Turner's syndrome", but autosomal dominant inheritance is frequent and the condition occurs in both sexes, although without any recognisable chromosomal abnormality. In common with Turner's syndrome, there is usually short stature and sometimes short neck with low hairline or neck webbing, abnormalities of the eyes (but commonly with ptosis, epicanthic folds, and anti-mongoloid slant), cubitus valgus, multiple small naevi, and defective nails. The facial appearance is characteristic with hypertelorism and a flat bridge to the nose, low set ears with atypical edges, and micrognathia. Cardiac abnormalities are common and the most serious implication of the condition, but of a different type to Turner's syndrome, involving the right ventricular outflow tract (pulmonary stenosis) and also atrial or ventricular septal defects or cardiomyopathy. Chest deformity is common, with depressed or elevated sternum and with widely spaced nipples. There is commonly mild mental retardation and sometimes defective hearing. Ovarian function, unlike in Turner's syndrome, is normal in girls, but boys commonly have undescended testes and may have delayed puberty. The adult height centile distribution is slightly higher than that of untreated Turner's syndrome. (See Case 18.)

Silver–Russell syndrome: this is one of the conditions of severe intrauterine growth retardation with continuing poor postnatal growth. The head is proportionately large, the face triangular, the mouth thin lipped with downturned corners, and micrognathia is common. Individuals are usually slender and underweight. There is a wide spectrum of additional features and those specifically described in the Silver syndrome include asymmetry due to underdevelopment of one side of the body or part of it, and precocious puberty, resulting in even shorter adult stature than would otherwise be expected. Motor development may be delayed but mental retardation is uncommon. Most cases are sporadic with no recognisable inheritance pattern. (See Case 19.)

Prader–Willi syndrome: this is a condition of poor growth associated with obesity, usually severe mental retardation and developmental delay, hypogonadism, and severe hypotonia in early life. The longitudinal growth pattern is characteristic, with poor weight gain and feeding difficulties in early childhood, but changing to progressive obesity and increased appetite after a few years as muscle strength improves. The obesity is more evident centrally than peripherally. There is, however, no acceleration in height, which usually remains at a low centile. Hands and feet are small. There is a characteristic facial appearance, with narrow forehead, almond shaped eyes and a triangular mouth. Hypogenitalism occurs in both sexes, with hypogonadism and infertility, scrotal hypoplasia, and cryptorchidism in boys, and poorly developed labia in girls. Initially the children are placid, but become increasingly demanding and difficult with major behavioural problems. Sex incidence is equal and about two thirds of cases have a demonstrable chromosome abnormality with a deletion on chromosome 15; the remainder are clinically similar but have normal chromosomes. (See Case 20.)

Conditions with Tall Stature

Non-pathological

Familial

As with short stature, the commonest cause of tall stature is that the parents are also tall. This effect may be temporarily exaggerated by the fact that tall children frequently go into puberty earlier than short children and by having their growth spurt earlier will accelerate at the time but will ultimately lose this extra height because they stop growing earlier. The effect of this timing of puberty is illustrated by Case 21, 22 and 23.

Exogenous obesity (Chapter 4, p. 43)

In contrast to endocrine causes of obesity which are associated with short stature, children with the commoner exogenous form of obesity tend to be tall. This is linked with an advancement of bone age and "physiological" age so that they frequently go through puberty at an earlier than average age and do not necessarily end up tall. (See Cases 24, 25 and 26.)

Pathological

Familial

The best recognised familial tall stature condition inherited as an autosomal dominant is Marfan's syndrome. Individuals with this condition have long thin fingers and toes (arachnodactyly), long limbs with reduced body upper to lower segment ratio, hypotonia and joint laxity, and a high arched palate. Complications are frequent, namely kyphoscoliosis, visual problems – notably subluxation or dislocation of the lens and myopia – and serious cardiovascular conditions, notably dilatation of the aorta and aortic valve and aortic aneurysms. (See Case 27.)

Endocrine

These conditions are uncommon in childhood (notably growth hormone excess – pituitary gigantism). Tallness is associated with advancement of bone age, and though reduction in ultimate stature might therefore be expected, this is clearly not inevitable and depends on the particular pathology, and the ages of onset of the condition and when treatment is instituted.

Examples:

Thyrotoxicosis, more frequent in girls than boys, is uncommon in childhood, but shows the typical features seen in adults, though with the additional component of accelerated growth. In view of this, weight loss is unlikely, but there is usually a reduction in the fat component and a fall in weight centile at a time when the height centile is rising. On treatment, height velocity and bone age advancement slow down and weight is regained. (See Case 28.)

Sexual precocity (see Chapter 6): whether precocious sexual development is due to true "central" puberty or to the abnormal production of sex hormones in excessive amounts not under pituitary gonadotrophin drive, height, weight, and bone age accelerate dramatically. The extent to which these can be slowed down with treatment and a reasonable ultimate height be achieved, depends on the cause, and the age and severity at the time of diagnosis. In many cases ultimate height will be reduced even with appropriate treatment. (See Cases 29, 30 and 31.)

Other conditions

Klinefelter's syndrome (47,XXY karyotype)   This condition is frequently not diagnosed until adult life, when investigations into infertility bring it to light. It is the commonest cause of infertility in men, accounting for 10% of cases. In childhood boys are frequently tall with proportionately long lower limbs. There may be no other diagnostic features at this time, though some, but by no means all, individuals are of below average intelligence, sometimes with disturbances of behaviour. The testes are small (less than 2 cm long in adulthood, incapable of producing viable sperm) but the degree of testosterone production at puberty is variable. Puberty is frequently delayed and secondary sexual characteristics may be poorly developed. Gynaecomastia occurs in about 40% of cases at a pubertal age and subsequently. (See Cases 32 and 33.)

47,XYY males   Boys with this condition are frequently tall, and end up as tall adults (average height 185 cm) but with normal body proportions. In the majority of cases there are no other clinical features and, as fertility is usually unimpaired, the abnormality will probably never be recognised. Intelligence is sometimes below average and most of these individuals have a low temper threshold becoming easily frustrated and irrational at such times, but in only a few is this a serious problem or behaviour irresponsible. There is a higher proportion of 47,XYY individuals reported in prisons and institutions for mentally subnormal males; the reasons for this are unclear as the majority are not aggressive, antisocial, or of low intelligence. (See Case 34.)

Sotos syndrome (cerebral gigantism)   Excessive growth, which usually begins before birth, is associated with accelerated skeletal and dental development. The facial appearance is unusual with high prominent fore-head (often with frontal baldness), hypertelorism and prognathism, large ears, and a large head circumference. Hands, feet, and sometimes genitalia are also large. Adult height is usually average, however, the accelerated growth rate slowing at around the end of the first decade. There is usually clumsiness, notably of fine motor movements, mild mental handicap, and retarded psychomotor development. Most cases are sporadic but there have been occasional reports of dominant inheritance. (See Case 35.)

Examples of growth disorders

In many of the illustrations, the age in decimal years is shown, as well as an arrow on the vertical height scale to represent the 50th centile for a child of that age and sex.

PSYCHOSOCIAL DEPRIVATION AND NEGLECT

1 This boy was referred at the age of $2\frac{1}{2}$ years because of poor growth. He had been of low birth weight, 2280 g at term, and had progressed poorly physically and developmentally, but was said to have had a good appetite. He had three older siblings, two with no problems, but one with similar stunting of growth. He was unresponsive, withdrawn, and miserable, playing with his hands and rocking. He was undernourished with scratched, dry skin, and was markedly retarded developmentally. Investigation revealed complete absence of growth hormone response to adequate insulin hypoglycaemia, but because of suspicions regarding his care he was not treated

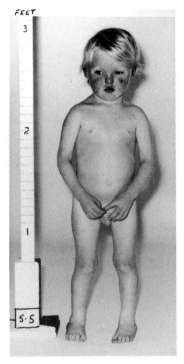

Case 1 at age 2·5 years

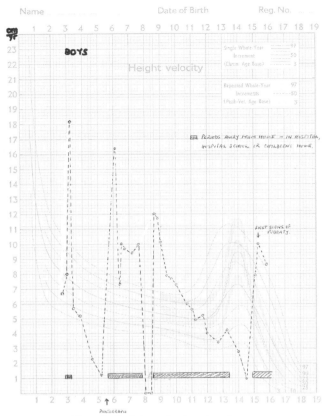

Case 1 (height velocity chart)

with growth hormone. After extensive social work input, case conferences, and so on, he was placed away from his home. The growth chart shows the dramatic changes in weight, height, and height velocity over the years on each occasion that he was away from home, with rapid recurrence of weight loss on returning to the home environment. These growth changes were paralleled by changes in temperament, wellbeing, and activity. Growth hormone production was normal when retested when in care. He remained away from home permanently from the age of $8\frac{1}{2}$ years and grew well, though markedly delayed in puberty. When last seen at 16·1 years he was still only in mid-puberty but with a height of 160·5 cm and considerable residual growth potential.

108

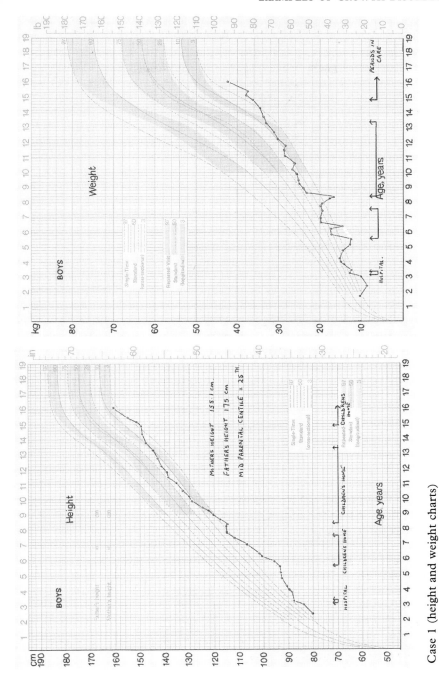

Case 1 (height and weight charts)

109

CHRONIC UPPER AIRWAY INFECTIONS AS CAUSE OF POOR APPETITE AND GROWTH

2 This boy grew well, with height and weight on the 50th centile until the age of 4 (mid-parental height centile was about the 40th). Subsequently he developed frequent upper respiratory infections and hay fever, and became fussy over food. The growth charts show the fall off in height and weight between ages 4 and 6 years. At the age of 6, tonsils and adenoids were removed with dramatic improvement in general health, food intake and growth.

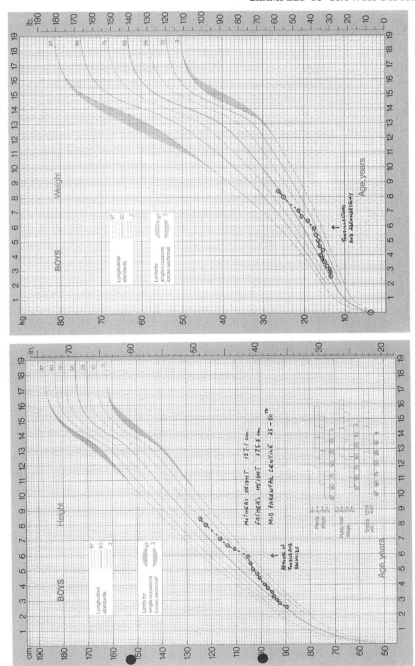

Case 2 (height and weight charts)

ANOREXIA NERVOSA

3 This basically healthy, intelligent girl had developed and grown normally until late adolescence with a height initially on the 90th centile, but because puberty was earlier than average (menarche age $12\frac{1}{4}$) full height was achieved at about 13 years on the 75th adult centile (just greater than the mid-parental centile). An older sister, rather plumper, had also reached the menarche early (age 11 years). Her father had died when the girl was 9 years old. Up until the age of $14\frac{1}{2}$ her weight had been satisfactory, approximating to the 50th centile, but then progressively fell, as shown in the weight chart on page 113 (and menstruation stopped at the age of 15). Initially no underlying problems were apparent, and it was not until nearly a year later, when her weight had fallen by 14 kg, that it became apparent that she was not eating adequately. She denied problems and maintained she was healthy and happy at school and fully active physically. Psychiatric assessment revealed that she was a girl with a rather obsessional personality, very dependent on her mother, and fearful of growing up. Fortunately the situation responded well to psychiatric counselling involving also her mother, and her weight was regained with resumption of menses after six months.

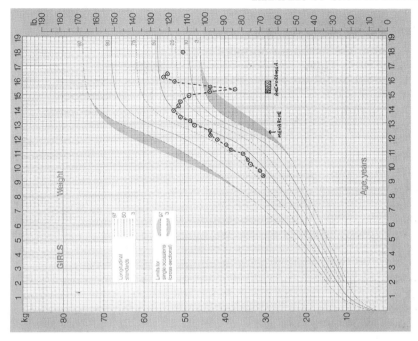

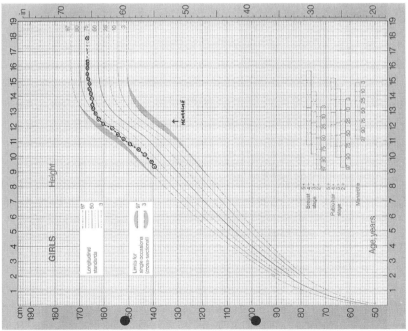

Case 3 (height and weight charts)

113

COELIAC DISEASE

4 This infant, the first born of dizygotic twin girls, birth weight 3800 g (the other twin having weighed 3400 g), presented at the age of 15 months with a three month history of having intermittent diarrhoea, and being miserable, irritable, and off her food, with recent vomiting and abdominal distension. Prior to weaning, her weight gain had been satisfactory, but as the centile chart shows, she had become grossly underweight, wasted, and in marked contrast to her twin sister. Jejunal biopsy confirmed the clinical diagnosis of coeliac disease, showing subtotal villous atrophy. (A paternal uncle also had coeliac disease.) She responded well to a gluten free diet (though for a period of three months she also required restriction of lactose because of transient secondary lactose intolerance). Growth and improvement in wellbeing were dramatic and after three months she had almost caught up with her twin sister. She remained on the gluten free diet and at the age of 13 was of height close to the 50th centile, identical to that of her twin, although 13 kg lighter in weight!

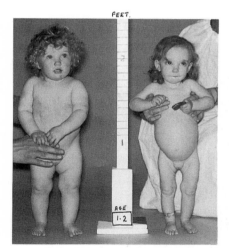 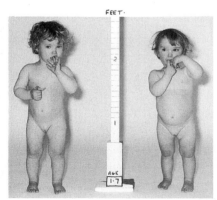

Case 4: before and 6 months after treatment, with twin sister on left

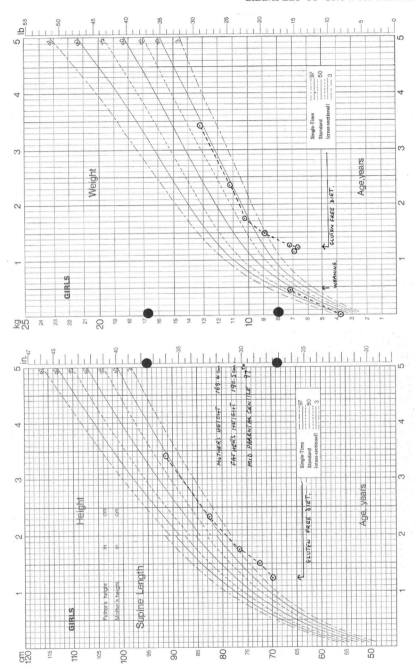

Case 4 (height and weight charts)

115

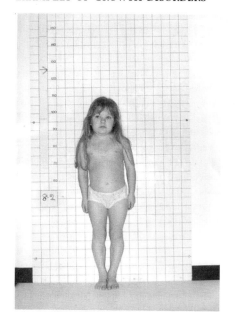 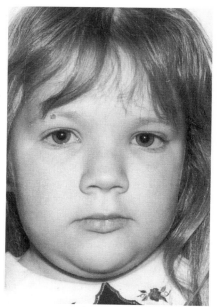

Case 5 at age 8·2 years

ACQUIRED HYPOTHYROIDISM

5 This girl presented at the age of $8\frac{1}{4}$ with a history of poor growth over the preceding year, but with no other symptoms, and her school performance was good. Birth weight at term had been 3070 g and earlier growth and development had been normal. Clinically she had a classically myxoedematous appearance, with a deep voice, slow pulse, and slowly relaxing tendon jerks. Bone age was retarded by three years. Testing confirmed primary hypothyroidism (but without thyroid antibodies) and she has responded well to treatment with thyroxine, initially 50 µg daily, gradually increasing to 100 µg over the years. She has been about a year later than average in her progress through puberty.

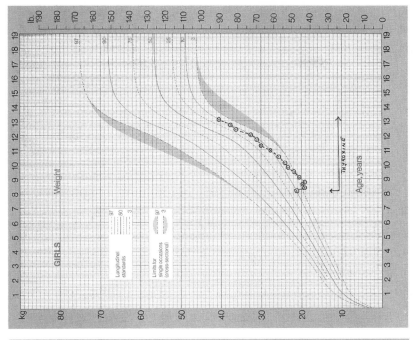

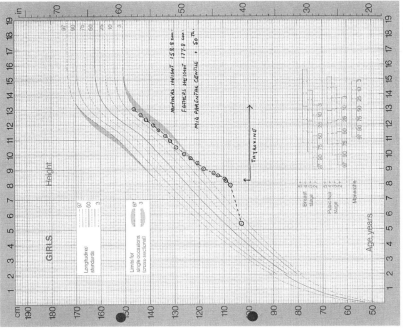

Case 5 (height and weight charts)

117

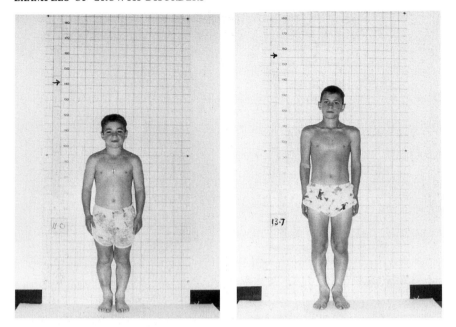

Case 6: before and after treatment

6 Past school records showed that the growth in height of this boy had been falling off for several years, though not his weight, so that at presentation at the age of 11 he was very short of stature and markedly overweight. The parents had not been concerned as they were also short of stature and his general health, activity, and school performance were good. Clinically he was muscular and short limbed, with a deep voice, bradycardia, and slowly relaxing tendon jerks. Tests confirmed severe primary hypothyroidism with positive thyroid antibodies, and he has responded well to doses of thyroxine, which have required progressive increase from 50 to 200 μg daily. Bone age at presentation was only a year retarded, but he was delayed in puberty, the first signs not appearing until 13. Subsequently progress in puberty was very rapid, and ultimate stature remained short.

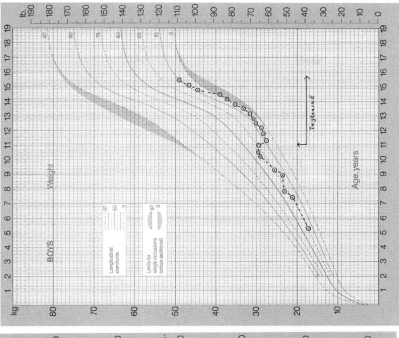

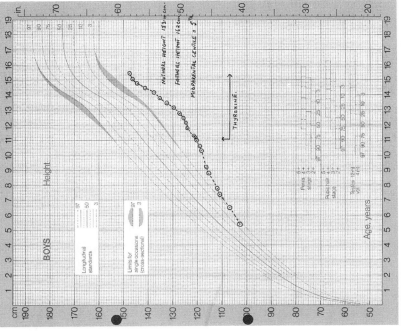

Case 6 (height and weight charts)

119

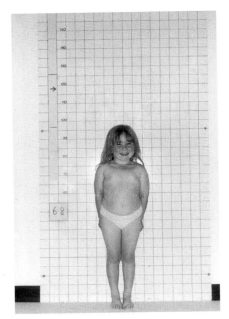

Case 7 before treatment at 6·8 years

GROWTH HORMONE DEFICIENCY

7 This 7 year old girl had been large at birth, weighing 3860 g. From the age of 18 months her growth had fallen off, height much more than weight, and she became obese. At the age of 3 she developed asthma and required regular inhaled steroid treatment from the age of $4\frac{1}{2}$, but not in growth suppressant dosage. Her development and health otherwise were good. Bone age at the age of 6·8 years corresponded to that of an average girl of 2·8 years. Investigations showed normal thyroid function but an almost total failure of response of growth hormone to stimulation.

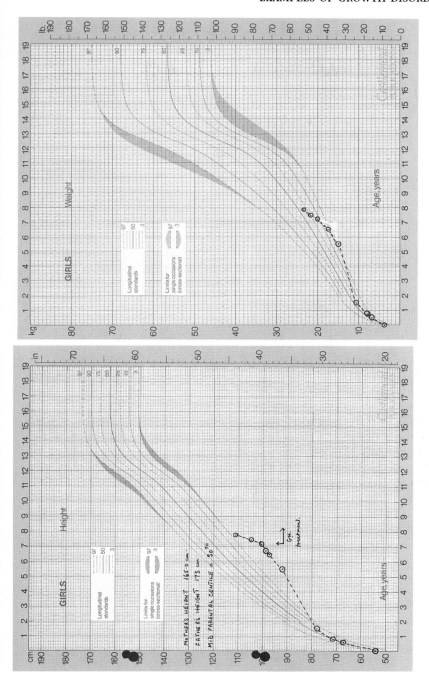

Case 7 (height and weight charts)

121

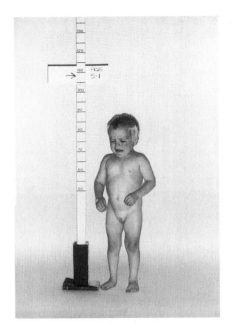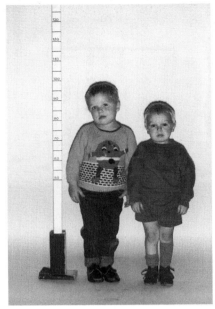

Case 8: with younger brother on left

8 This boy is pictured at the age of 5·1 years with his brother who at age 4 years was 9 cm taller. He had been large at birth, weighing 4430 g, but his growth appeared to fall off from the age of about 2 years. He had been a little late in developmental milestones, particularly with speech, but his general health had been good. At presentation he was very short, moderately obese, and had small genitalia. Bone age was two years retarded. Testing showed complete absence of growth hormone, but normal thyroid function. He has shown a reasonable response to treatment with growth hormone with a very dramatic initial reduction in skinfold measurements.

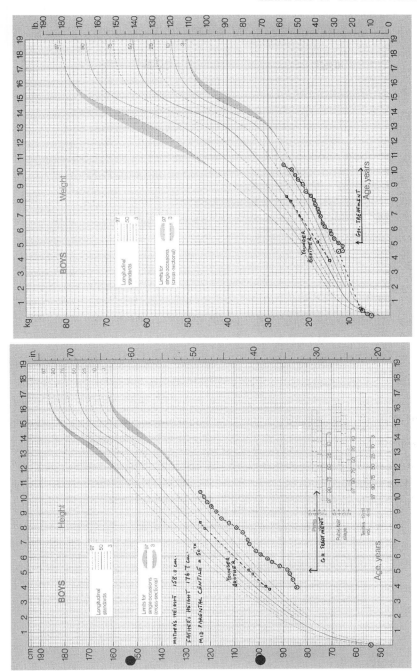

Case 8 (height and weight charts)

123

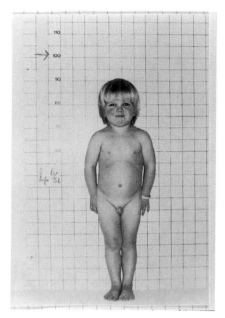

Case 9 before treatment at 4·2 years

PANHYPOPITUITARISM

9 Concern about the the extreme short stature of this boy was not expressed until he had reached the age of nearly $3\frac{1}{2}$. He had been a good size at birth, weighing 3400 g at 36 weeks gestation, but had been born by breech delivery and had had prolonged neonatal jaundice which, though relatively mild, had persisted for two months. At the age of 2 he had been unconscious for five minutes following a head injury, but his early life, apart from poor growth, had been otherwise uneventful and his developmental progress had been normal. Initial investigation showed secondary hypothyroidism and fuller studies were delayed until this had been treated. He was then shown to have growth hormone deficiency (though with a good cortisol response to insulin hypo-glycaemia) and when tested at a later age proved also to be gonadotrophin deficient. Though having a rather excessive thirst and polyuria, this was shown not to be due to diabetes insipidus. No underlying cause for the hypopituitarism was identified. Bone age at the age of 5 years when growth hormone treatment was started was that of an average boy of $3\frac{1}{4}$ years.

124

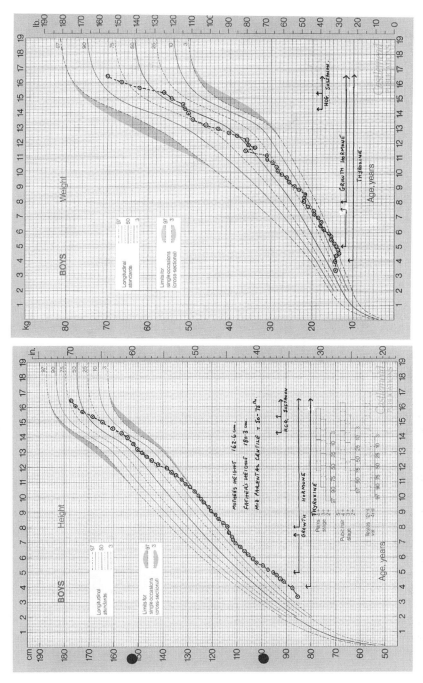

Case 9 (height and weight charts)

125

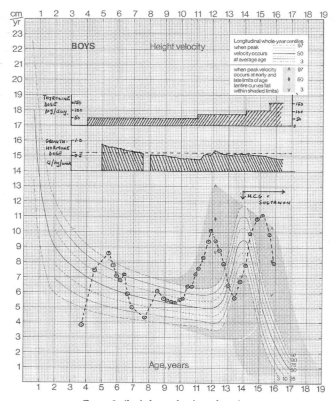

Case 9 (height velocity chart)

His response to treatment has been interesting, as shown on his height velocity chart. During the time of treatment with human growth hormone and the early period after the introduction of biosynthetic hormone, dosage was standard irrespective of age and size, that is, four units three times weekly. In the light of subsequent recommendations (0·6 units/kg/week) this had resulted in young children having a large dose which became progressively less on a weight for weight basis as they grew older. This boy's chart illustrates the relationship of the height velocity to dosage (and also that there was a marked reduction in velocity over the six month period when human growth hormone was withdrawn). When the dosage of biosynthetic growth hormone was increased in accordance with new recommendations (when he was at an age of about 11) there was a dramatic increase in velocity which was not linked with puberty.

126

Being gonadotrophin deficient, puberty required hormone treatment (initially with human chorionic gonadotrophin, subsequently with Sustanon) which was initiated at the age of 14. Despite the growth hormone dosage being rather low at this stage, the height velocity through puberty has been dramatic and this young man's ultimate stature is well up to expectations on the basis of mid-parental height centiles and those of his siblings.

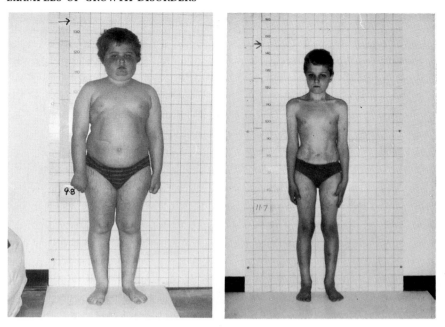

Case 10: on steroid treatment and after withdrawal

GLUCOCORTICOID EXCESS

10 At the age of 1·2 years this boy was diagnosed as having an as-trocytoma, for which (following the insertion of a ventriculo–peritoneal shunt for obstructive hydrocephalus) he was treated with cranial ir-radiation and steroids. For six years he made good progress and grew satisfactorily, and during this time endocrine investigation showed nor-mal hypothalamic–pituitary function. At the age of $8\frac{1}{2}$ years he developed a recurrence of the tumour which was treated with (among other things) high dose dexamethasone for nearly two years. Over this period his growth in height became very slow, with enormous weight gain, and the development of very obvious Cushingoid features, as illustrated in the photographs taken at the age of 9·8 years. Following gradual cessation of the steroid treatment, his normal growth rate resumed and his weight fell without any hormone or other treatment.

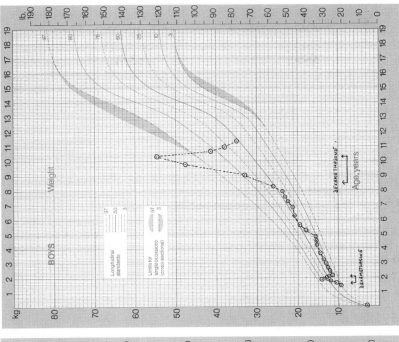

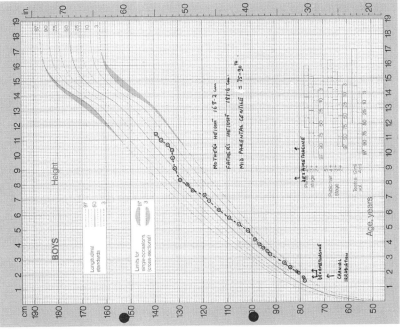

Case 10 (height and weight charts)

11 This boy, though diagnosed as having asthma from infancy, was not actively treated until the age of 6, when he was given inhaled steroids, the dose being progressively increased over the course of a year. He had been a large baby at birth, weighing 3900 g, and had grown satisfactorily over the early years. As well as having asthma, he suffered from hay fever and showed many other allergic features. From the age of 7 he was lost to hospital follow up for two years, during which time he continued on inhaled budesonide in a total daily dosage of 800 µg. During this time his height centile fell from between the 25th and 50th to just below the 10th, and at the age of 9 his bone age was retarded by 2·3 years. Over this period he had been relatively free from symptoms of asthma, and it was possible to halve his inhaled steroid dosage without deterioration in the asthma and with consequent improved height velocity. In situations like this, poor growth could be due either to poor control of the disease, or to the effects of excessive treatment, and in this case the latter was much the more likely.

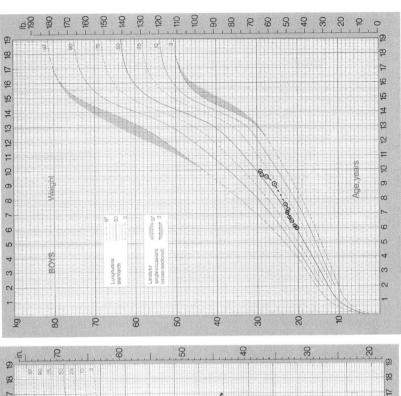

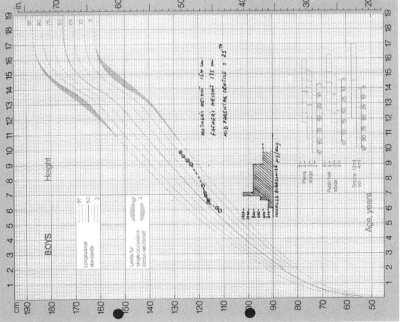

Case 11 (height and weight charts)

131

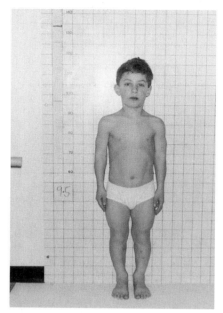

Case 12 at 9·5 years

BONE DYSPLASIAS

Achondroplasia

12 This boy had been a good size at birth, weighing 4200 g at term, and had parents of above average stature. It was not until 15 months of age that the health visitor noticed that he was short of stature when walking, and appeared overweight, this actually being due to the body disproportion because his limbs were markedly short in relation to a more normal size trunk and head. Radiographic studies confirmed the diagnosis of achondroplasia. His general health, development, activity, and intellect were normal. At the age of 10 he underwent surgical leg lengthening procedures with an increase in stature of about 8 cm. In this example, as in the majority of cases, the condition was due to new mutation.

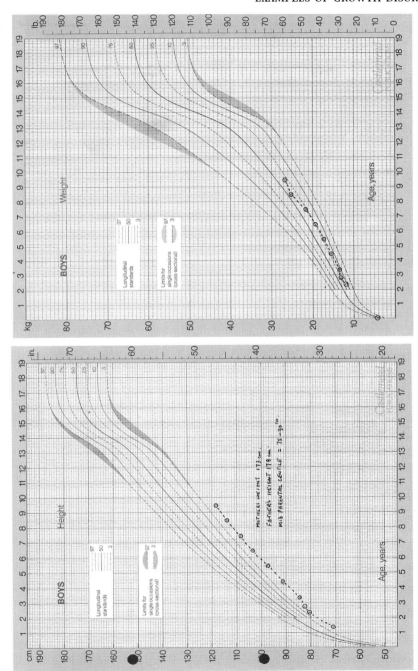

Case 12 (height and weight charts)

133

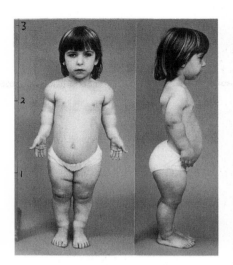
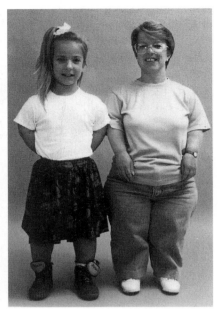

Case 13: at 6·3 years and at 12·5 years with her mother

13 This girl, whose mother is achondroplastic, shows the classic features of the condition. Her birth weight was 3040 g and she was born by elective caesarian section. According to the centile standards she was always overweight, and although initially this was largely due to the effects of body disproportion, she has also become obese. She is going to be rather taller as an adult than her mother (influenced by the tall stature of her father). She progressed through puberty at an early age, showing only a modest increase in height velocity at that time, and reached the menarche at 12. She declined surgery for leg lengthening and is quite content with her short stature.

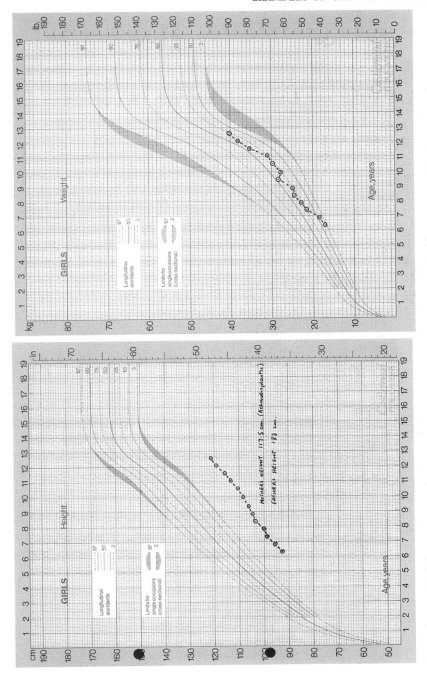

Case 13 (height and weight charts)

135

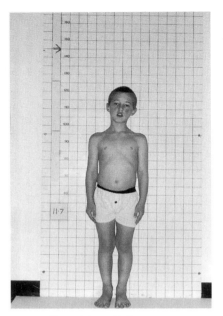

Case 14 at 11·7 years

Dyschondro-osteosis

14 This boy probably has a milder form of bone dysplasia, which like many others is not clinically obvious. He had been a good size at birth, weighing 3570 g at term. Development and general health have been normal, but his growth was poor from an early stage, with his weight always at a higher centile than his height. Body proportions showed the shortness to be more evident in the limbs. Endocrine investigations did not show any hormonal deficiency, and bone age has been appropriate for his actual age throughout. Subtle changes seen on radiographs have suggested the diagnosis of this rare bone dysplasia.

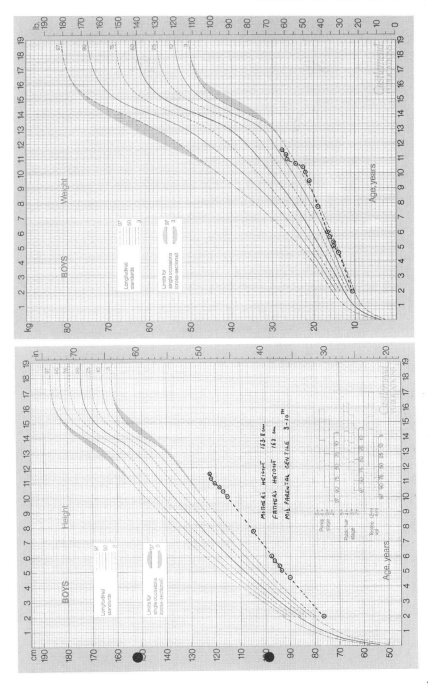

Case 14 (height and weight charts)

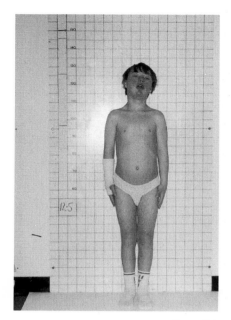 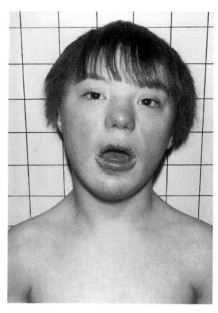

Case 15 at 12·5 years

DOWN'S SYNDROME

15 This boy, with typical features of Down's syndrome (and karyotype 47,XY with trisomy 21) has had poor growth from birth (birth weight 2660 g at full term), probably made worse by having severe congenital heart disease (atrioventricular canal defect). During the first five years of life he had recurrent chest infections and episodes of congestive cardiac failure, but has had less trouble since that time and is maintained on treatment with digoxin and diuretics. Endocrine function throughout has been normal and bone age appropriate for chronological age.

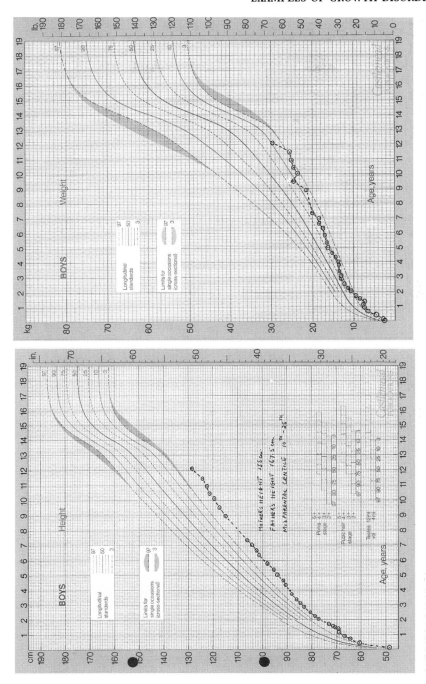

Case 15 (height and weight charts)

TURNER'S SYNDROME

16 One of these twins has Turner's syndrome (karyotype 46,XX 45, XO mosaic), the other being normal; the adverse effect of the condition on growth is evidenced by comparison of their centile charts. They were born at term, with birth weight of the girl with Turner's syndrome being 2600 g and that of her twin sister 2800 g. The characteristic features of Turner's syndrome shown, in addition to the poor growth, are the extreme web neck and high arched palate. She also had mild aortic stenosis. At the age of $5\frac{1}{2}$ years treatment was started with growth hormone, with dramatic improvement in height velocity, so that after two years the height difference between the girls, initially 9 cm, had fallen to 1·6 cm. However, this had been linked with a very rapid advancement of bone age, which had been commensurate with actual age at the start of treatment at $5\frac{1}{2}$ but by the age of 7 was $2\frac{1}{4}$ years advanced. At the age of 8 the response to growth hormone stopped (possibly due to the development of growth hormone antibodies) and growth remained at only 2·5 cm per year over nearly two years of further treatment. Treatment has now been discontinued. The sister's growth has remained consistent throughout with height close to the 50th centile (without treatment) and she is again becoming progressively the taller.

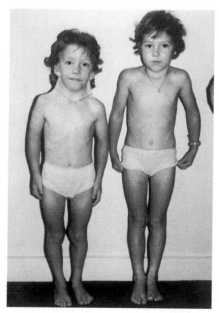

Case 16 with twin sister on the right at 5·5 years

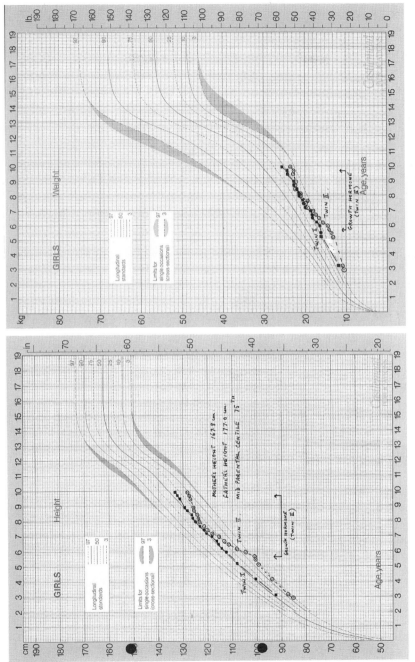

Case 16 with twin (height and weight charts)

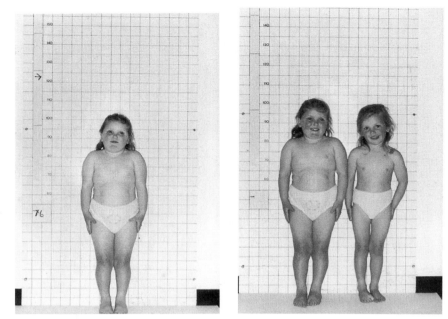

Case 17: with sister, 3 years younger, on the right

17 In contrast to the case history above, this short statured girl showed no clinical features suggestive of Turner's syndrome. The chromosomal abnormality is complex, with one normal X chromosome and one isodicentric X chromosome made up of two copies of the long arm of an X, that is, trisomic for the long arm of the X, and monosomic for the short arm. The girl had become markedly overweight through early childhood and the only clinical feature in keeping with the diagnosis was recurrent middle ear infections (requiring insertion of grommets). Treatment with growth hormone from $8\frac{1}{4}$ years of age, although accompanied by dramatic initial weight loss, resulted in only a trivial change in height velocity. Bone age throughout has been commensurate with calendar age, and other investigations of endocrine function have been normal. The illustration shows her with her sister, who is 3 years younger.

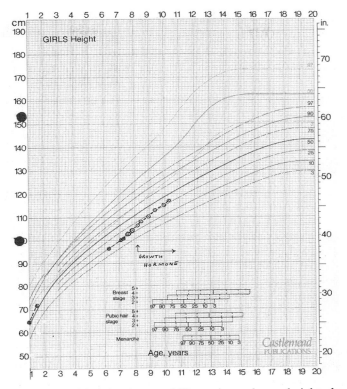

Case 17 (standard height chart and Turner's syndrome height chart)

NOONAN'S SYNDROME

18 This sister and brother both have normal karyotypes, and this clearly represents a familial case of Noonan's syndrome with the father and his two children showing the typical phenotype and short stature. Both father and son had bilateral testicular maldescent requiring surgery. Both children suffer from profound sensorineural deafness, attending a special school for the deaf. Both children were born after normal pregnancies, the daughter weighing 2360 g at 36 weeks gestation, and her brother 2750 g at 38 weeks.

The girl's height throughout has followed a course just above the third centile and weight close to this. She had the classical facial appearance, in addition to mild neck webbing and shortening with a low posterior hair line. She had joint hypermobility, bilateral fifth finger clinodactyly, and a mild degree of cubitus valgus.

Her brother had a similar growth pattern, with height running just below the third centile, but parallel to it. He had pectus excavatum, with a shield shaped chest and widely spaced nipples. Both testes were incompletely descended, lying high in the inguinal canal. He, too, had joint hypermobility, bilateral fifth finger clinodactyly, and mild cubitus valgus. As well as the classical facial appearance of Noonan's syndrome, with hypertelorism and low set abnormally shaped prominent ears, he had mild neck webbing and shortening, but the hair line was not low.

Their father had mild neck webbing, low posterior hairline, pectus excavatum, cubitus valgus, bilateral ptosis with hypertelorism, and low set ears.

Echocardiograms performed on the father and children were normal at this stage. Endocrine investigations were normal in both children, and bone ages commensurate with their actual ages.

144

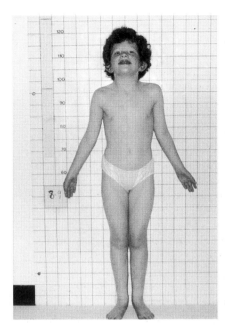

Case 18a at 8·9 years

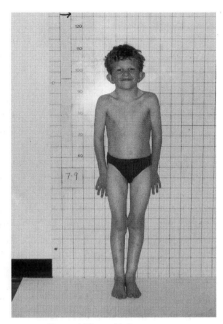

Case 18b at 7·9 years

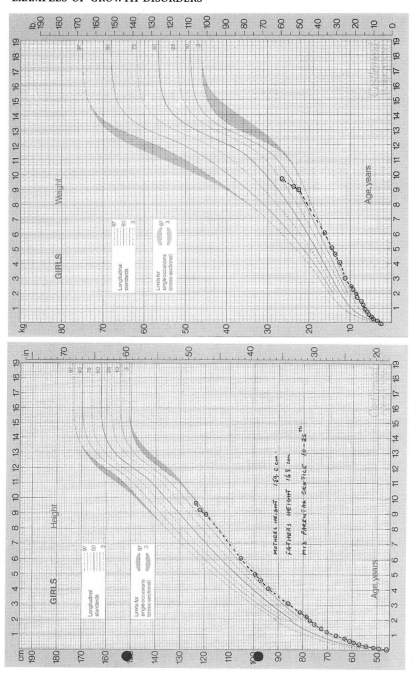

Case 18 (a) (height and weight charts)

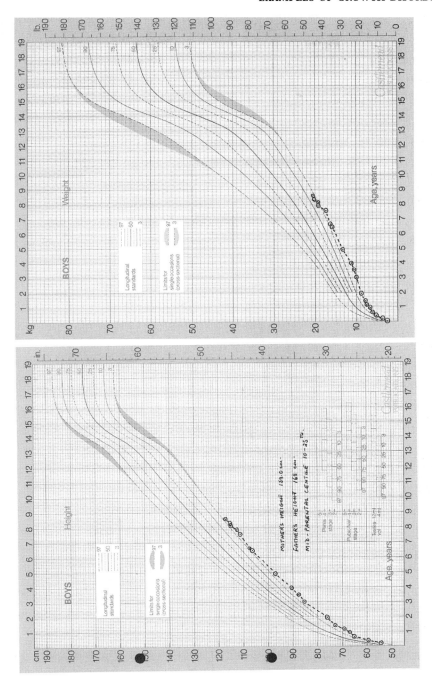

Case 18 (b) (height and weight charts)

147

SILVER-RUSSELL SYNDROME

19 This boy was very small at birth, weighing only 1850 g at term following an uneventful pregnancy, and also short in length. He has remained small without any progressive fall away, and his weight has been throughout at a much lower centile than height. He has the characteristic appearance of this condition, with triangular face and marked asymmetry of the body, the right leg being 2·5 cm shorter than the left and much smaller also in girth. His intellectual development has been normal throughout. Endocrine function has been normal but bone age is retarded by about two years.

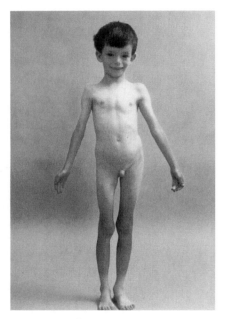

Case 19

PRADER-WILLI SYNDROME

20 This boy was somewhat light for dates at birth, weighing 2070 g at 36 weeks gestation, delivery having been induced because of low maternal oestriols and poor growth in the final month. He was a very floppy infant with difficulty swallowing and poor initial weight gain. He had undescended testes and underdeveloped genitalia. His subsequent development was only mildly delayed, and at the age of $2\frac{1}{2}$ years his

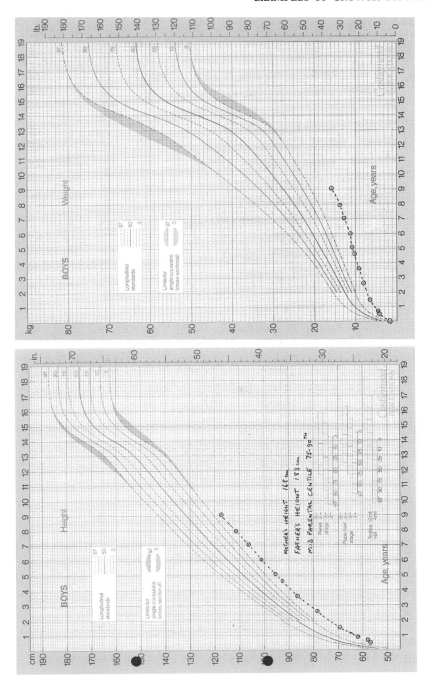

Case 19 (height and weight charts)

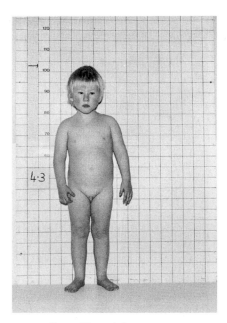

Case 20 at 4·3 years

developmental quotient (Griffiths) was 85, with more difficulties in locomotor skills and eye–hand coordination than in other aspects. Speech was delayed and of nasal quality, possibly because of a very high palate. By the age of 4 (when the photograph was taken) he had the classical facial appearance of a child with Prader–Willi syndrome and with strabismus. He was not of short stature but beginning to show truncal obesity. The diagnosis was confirmed by karyotype showing a small deletion of the short arm of one of the number 15 chromosomes. From that age onwards, although his height adhered to the 25th centile, his appetite improved (ultimately becoming very difficult to control) and the weight gain increased disproportionately so that ultimately he became grossly overweight.

He progressed through normal school, but with difficulty and requiring extra help, and developed behavioural problems and temper tantrums. Both testes required orchidopexy, the left being intraperitoneal. He progressed through puberty at an average age, but without showing a normal pubertal growth spurt, and in consequence has ended up with an adult stature below the third centile.

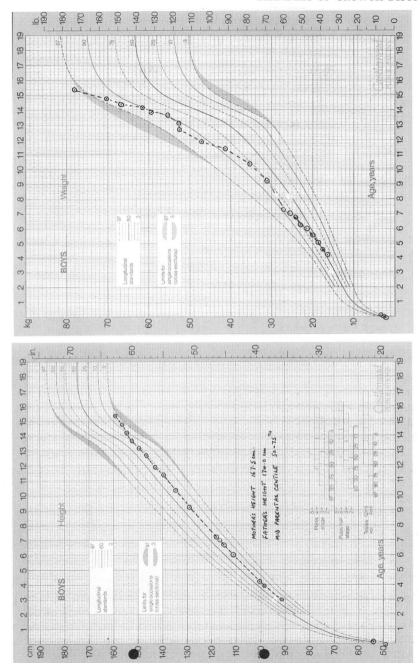

Case 20 (height and weight charts)

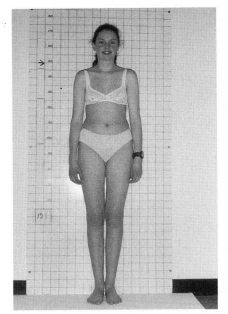

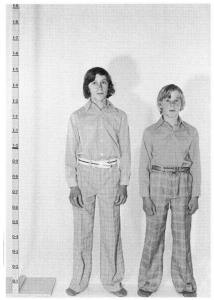

Case 21 at 12·1 years   Case 22 (a) + (b) at 14 years

FAMILIAL TALL STATURE

21 This very tall girl has been large from birth (weighing 3690 g at term). She entered puberty early, and between the ages of 9 and 10 her height increased by 12·5 cm and her weight by 11 kg. At the age of 10 her height was 14 cm above the 97th centile, but her bone age was nearly three years advanced. In consequence of this early growth spurt she reached the menarche at an age of just less than 11, and her growth rate then rapidly declined. It is apparent that she will effectively reach full stature by the age of 13, and this will be only slightly above the 97th centile for an adult woman.

Her mother, too, had been an early developer, reaching the menarche at the age of $9\frac{1}{2}$. This girl's father, himself 194 cm tall, came from a very tall family: his own father, who was over 192 cm tall, had a father and six brothers all between 187 cm and 200 cm tall, and three sisters over 183 cm in height.

ATYPICAL TIMING OF PUBERTY

22 Two dizygotic twin boys were of similar height before puberty and as adults, but of considerable difference in height at the age of about 14 because the one went into puberty much earlier than the other.

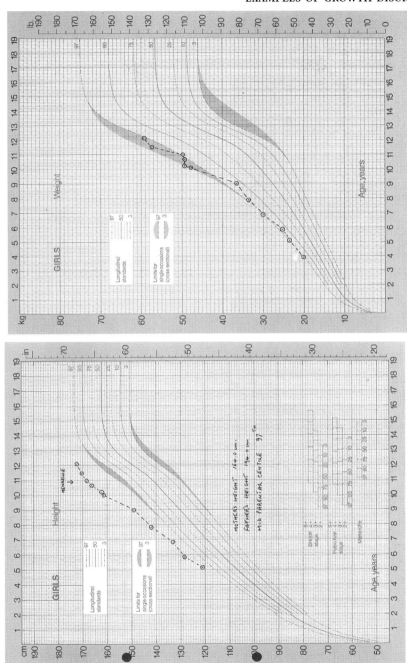

Case 21 (height and weight charts)

153

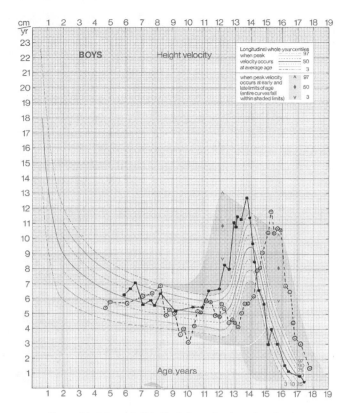

Case 23 (a) and (b) (height velocity chart)

23 The height and height velocities are shown of two brothers, one developing much earlier than the other. Having both been on the 50th centile for height before puberty, there was a 15 cm difference at the age of 14, yet ultimately the one shorter at that age ended up the taller as an adult.

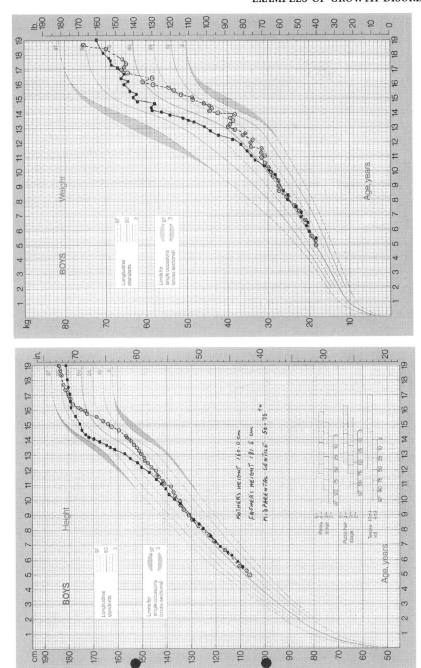

Case 23 (a) and (b) (height and weight charts)

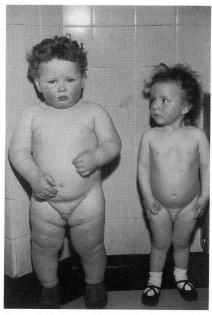

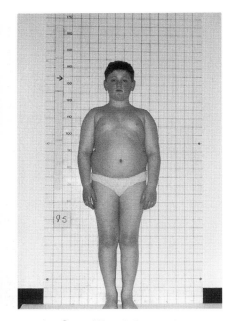

Case 24   Case 25 at 9·5 years

EXOGENOUS OBESITY

24 Fat and thin 2 year old boys are compared, the former showing an increase in all body proportions as well as just fatty tissue. The appearance of underdeveloped genitals is misleading because they are buried in fatty tissue.

25 Though not large at birth, weighing 3180 g at term, this boy became fat at an early age, with a huge appetite. The mid-parental height centile was between the 10th and 25th, the mother being 155 cm tall and the father 170 cm, but surprisingly neither was overweight. At the age of $9\frac{1}{2}$ the boy's weight was 53·0 kg, way above the 97th centile, but he was also 143 cm tall (between the 90th and 97th centiles) and with a bone age advanced at 10·8 years.

26 This girl was large at birth, weighing 4060 g at term. While being exclusively breast fed until 6 months, her weight gain had been reasonable, but from the time of weaning she gained weight excessively, despite apparently not overeating. When referred at the age of 5·8 years

156

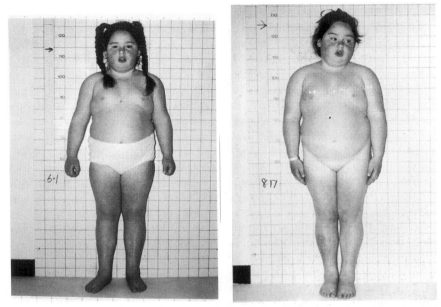

Case 26 at presentation at 6·1 years (left) and at 8·2 years when hypothyroid (right)

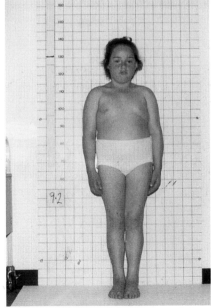

After treatment with thyroxine at 9·2 years

(Figure 26a), she had features strongly suggestive of exogenous, non-pathological, obesity, being also very tall and with a bone age advanced by two years. Attempts at dietary control over eight months were not very successful. She was referred back at the age of 8 (Figure 26b), after a further eighteen months, because of continuing weight gain despite rigid dieting. It was apparent, however, that over this period, despite the weight gain, height velocity had fallen drastically. Apart from some swelling of the ankles, there were no significant clinical features. Investigation showed that she had become severely *hypothyroid* (with positive thyroid antibodies). Bone age advancement had markedly slowed down (having increased by only 0·9 years in 2·2 years). Treatment with thyroxine resulted in a rapid fall in weight and acceleration in height velocity (Figure 26c). The primary problem of obesity, however, still exists, though to a lesser degree, and skinfold measurements are much less than at earlier stages. Puberty occurred at a slightly earlier than average age and the menarche was reached at the age of 12·6 years. Ultimate height was greater than expected on the basis of parental heights.

This case illustrates the importance of recognising that pathologies can develop in exogenously obese individuals, and of not being tied by rules of thumb, for example, that there is unlikely to be a pathology in tall, fat, growing children.

158

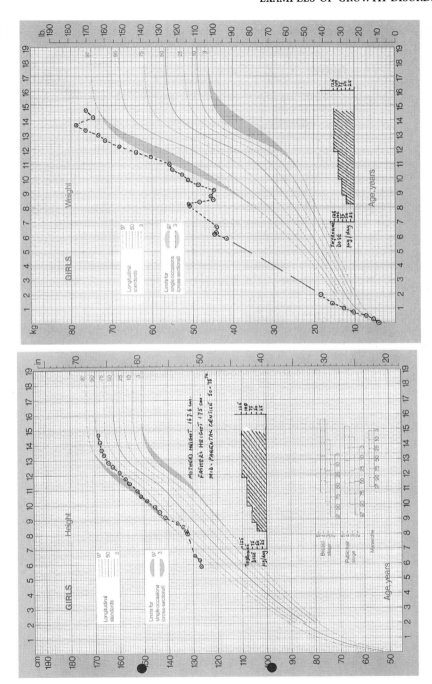

Case 26 (height and weight charts)

MARFAN'S SYNDROME

27 These sisters are descended from a family in which Marfan's syndrome has been present for at least three previous generations (see figure opposite). Their father had dislocated lenses and, having had an aortic valve replacement, died at the age of 33 from a dissecting aortic aneurysm.

Both girls are tall and thin, with long fingers and toes, hyperextensible joints, and high arched palates. The elder (Case 27b) had a birth weight of 3470 g at term and was tall from an early age. However, her bone age was about a year advanced throughout and she entered puberty at an early age, reaching the menarche at 12, and ultimate stature should not exceed 180 cm. She has myopia, but thus far shows no evidence of lens dislocation, nor does she have a cardiovascular or spinal abnormality, though she does have a mild chest deformity with a prominent lower sternum.

The younger sister, although a little larger at birth (weight 3800 g at term) has subsequently been slightly less tall at comparable ages. Her bone age, too, has been about a year advanced, giving a prediction for adult height slightly less than that of her sister. She has mitral valve prolapse, but no abnormality of the aorta or aortic valve. She required glasses from the age of 3 for progressive myopia, showed the first signs of lens slipping at the age of 4, and subsequently marked dislocation. She has also developed progressive lumbar scoliosis from the age of 6.

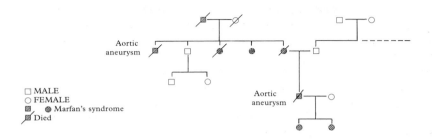

Aortic
aneurysm

☐ MALE
○ FEMALE
▨ ◉ Marfan's syndrome
▨ Died

Aortic
aneurysm

Case 27: family tree

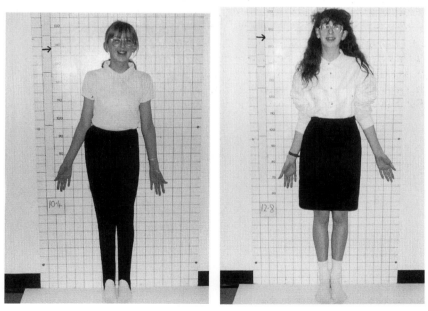

Case 27a   Case 27b

161

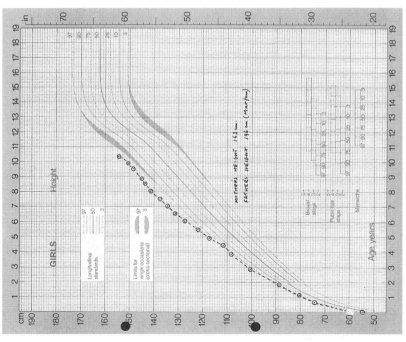

162

Case 27a (height and weight charts)

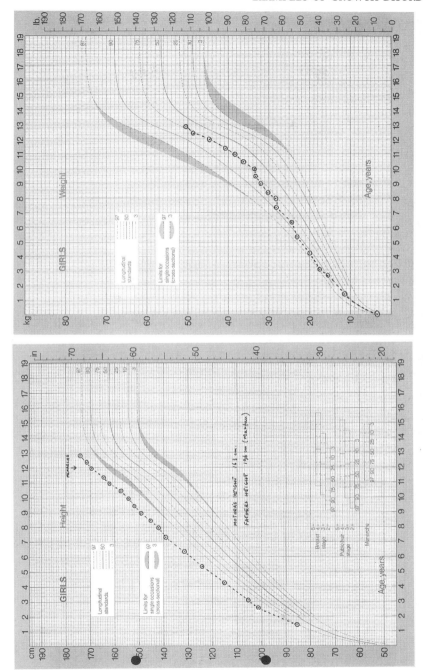

Case 27b (height and weight charts)

163

THYROTOXICOSIS

28 This boy presented at the age of $5\frac{1}{2}$, having previously had an uneventful history (birth weight 3530 g). For six months there had been an apparent progressive bulging of the eyes, and rapid growth without significant weight gain. He was rather lacking in energy, but fidgety and with a mild tremor, though no other thyrotoxic symptoms were reported. There was no family history of thyroid disease. On examination there was an impression of symmetrical exophthalmus, mainly produced by lid retraction. The thyroid was slightly diffusely enlarged, with a bruit, and there was a marked tachycardia. His height was just above the 97th centile, weight on the 90th (but subsequent progression indicated that this must have been considerably below his "norm"). Investigations showed very high circulating thyroid hormone levels, suppressed thyroid stimulating hormone and positive thyroid antibodies, confirming the diagnosis of Grave's disease. On treatment with carbimazole, he rapidly became euthyroid and gained weight, which over subsequent years has continued to progress irrevocably, his height having maintained a position on the 97th centile. At presentation his bone age was markedly advanced, being 9·0 years at an actual age of 5·3 years, and it has subsequently remained advanced despite his being maintained euthyroid, and the most recent estimate at an age of 10·2 years was 14·7 despite not yet being in puberty. This advancement is presumably the effect of severe "exogenous" obesity, which would appear to be familial in view of his parents' gross overweight.

The treatment was gradually tailed off and stopped without subsequent relapse after $2\frac{1}{2}$ years.

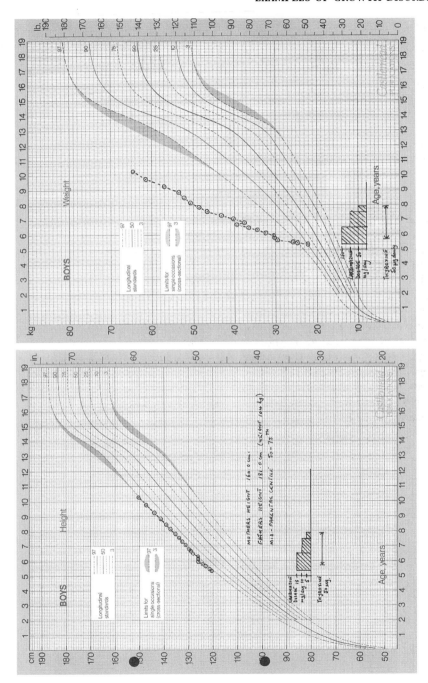

Case 28 (height and weight charts)

165

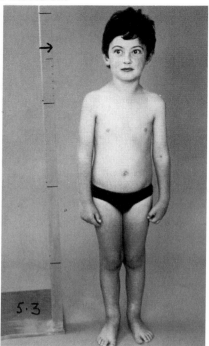

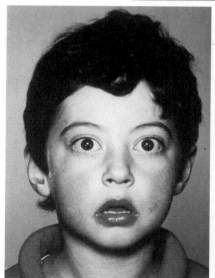
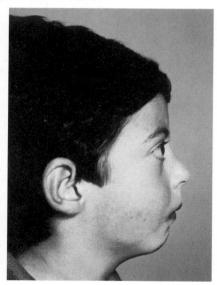

Case 28 at 5·3 years

PRECOCIOUS PUBERTY

29 These monozygotic boy twins both have neurofibromatosis with many cafe au lait patches, and were moderately delayed developmentally. Neither parent has the condition, which has presumably arisen by a new mutation. They were referred at the age of 5. From the age of $3\frac{1}{2}$ the first and bigger twin (birthweight 3150 g at term) showed rapid growth in height and weight and became very muscular. The second twin (birth weight 2780 g) also was growing faster than average, but to a lesser extent. For some time both boys were recognised as having greatly reduced visual acuity, and ophthalmoscopy showed bilateral optic atrophy. For six months prior to presentation, the first twin was showing pubertal changes, with genital and testicular growth, pubic hair, and offensive perspiration. The smaller twin did not show these features, but both had become overactive and excitable, and the larger twin in particular aggressive and disobedient. The bone age of the first twin was markedly advanced, being 9·7 years at an age of 5·1, and investigations revealed high gonadotrophin levels, confirming that he had central precocious puberty. Despite the lack of any physical features of puberty, the second twin also showed a degree of bone age advancement (6·6 years) and slight increase in gonadotrophins. At no stage did either twin show any other abnormality of endocrine function.

Computed tomography showed that both twins had masses in the suprasellar region, shown by biopsy in the larger twin to be a glioma of the optic chiasma with infiltration of both optic nerves. Both twins were treated with a five week course of cranial irradiation.

Treatment to control the pubertal process was started in the first twin with cyproterone acetate. This held the features of puberty in check, and improved the behaviour and body odour. His rapid growth persisted, however, and bone age continued to advance, so that he was effectively fully grown with fused epiphyses by the age of $11\frac{1}{2}$, with a height of only 155 cm.

Despite the lack of clinical features of puberty (which did not become evident until the age of $9\frac{1}{2}$) and with no acceleration of growth, the smaller twin had a rapidly advancing bone age, which at a chronological age of 6·6 years had reached that of an average boy of 9·2 years, and at 7 years of age offensive perspiration was apparent, so he was also started on cyproterone treatment. This was continued in both twins to the age of 11. At that age (when his brother was almost fully grown) the second twin was only showing the earliest clinical signs of puberty, yet his bone age was almost adult, and disappointingly he subsequently grew very little. It is surprising that he should have ended up the shorter of the

167

two, despite in the early stages having less evidence of precocious puberty and bone age advancement. Although the boys are monozygotic twins their physiques are different, and though both are of big build and overweight, this is more evident in the elder twin.

Sadly, vision has deteriorated, notably in the smaller twin who has become almost blind, but both progressed well in other respects without further treatment (and no evidence on computed tomography of progression in the tumour size) and are doing well in a school for the partially sighted.

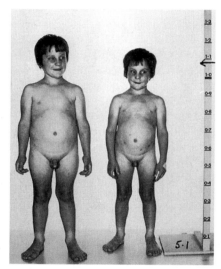

Case 29 (a) and (b) at 5·1 years

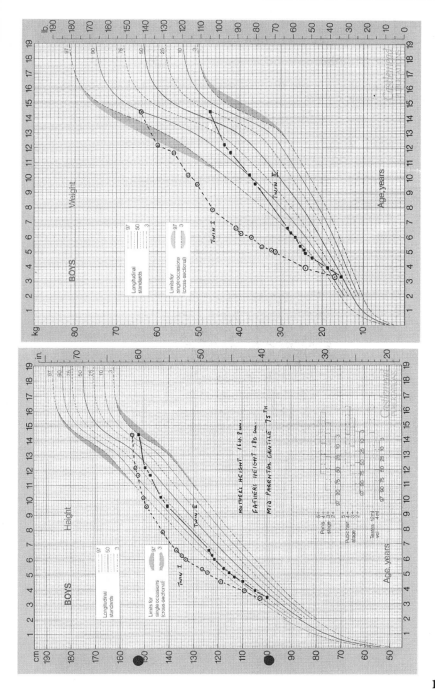

Case 29 (a) and (b) (height and weight charts)

30 Sexual precocity was evident in this boy before the age of 2. He had been large at birth, weighing 4125 g at term, and was noted then to have a large penis. His length had followed the 90th centile, appropriate for the family, until the age of 1 year, and then both length and weight diverged upwards. Between the ages of 1 and 2 years he developed pubic hair, a deep voice, and facial acne. He became strong and muscular and by the age of 2 years had a penis of almost adult size, experiencing frequent erections, yet the testes remained infantile in size. His behaviour was aggressive, and he showed inappropriate affection to all of the female sex. Extensive investigation showed the only biochemical abnormality to be a marked elevation of plasma testosterone (with low gonadotrophins) and this was shown to be testicular in origin. His bone age at 2 years of age was that of a 9 year old boy.

Owing to the problems in making a diagnosis, treatment was delayed until the age of 2·7 years when the boy was given ketoconazole, a drug which blocks steroid synthesis (he therefore also required cortisone replacement). This treatment rapidly resulted in improvement in behaviour, regression in the pubertal features, and slowing down of growth rate and bone age advancement; at the age of 6 years he had a bone age of a $12\frac{1}{2}$ year old. The dosage of ketoconazole has been progressively increased to maintain suppression of testosterone levels.

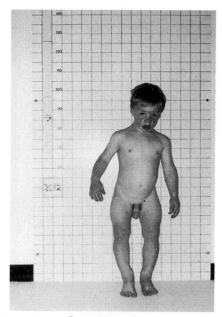

Case 30: at 2 years

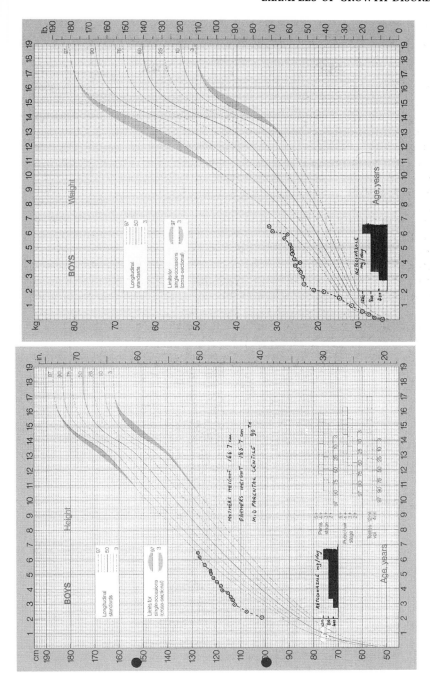

Case 30 (height and weight charts)

171

This condition, "testotoxicosis", which is due to a premature non-gonadotrophin dependent overactivity of the testosterone producing cells of the testes, though very rare, illustrates well the features of sexual precocity not central in origin, and particularly with regard to growth. A similar clinical picture is found if excessive androgen is produced by the adrenal glands, as in late presenting congenital adrenal hyperplasia or adrenal tumours.

31 At the age of $6\frac{1}{2}$ this girl first showed slight breast enlargement, but there was no acceleration of growth and bone age was appropriate. Two years later there had been a gradual progress in breast size and the start of pubic hair growth. Her height had accelerated a little and bone age was now a year advanced. The family declined treatment and the features of puberty continued to progress with the menarche at the age of $10\frac{1}{2}$, by which time height had risen to above the 90th centile and bone age was that of an average girl of just over 13 years. From that time growth slowed rapidly with a further increment of only 7 cm in height, adult height being only 154 cm (10th centile). She had shown a similar growth pattern to that of her mother, who was only 151 cm tall, having reached the menarche at the age of 11.

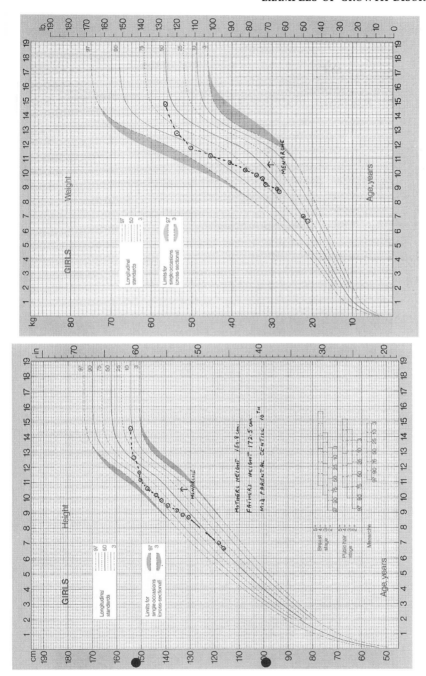

Case 31 (height and weight charts)

KLINEFELTER'S SYNDROME

32 This boy, of average birth weight at term (3300 g), developed seizures at the age of 5 months and was treated with phenobarbitone for three years, though having no further fits after the age of 14 months. His early milestones had been mildly retarded and he subsequently had learning difficulties at school, although he coped in a normal school with help. From the start he had been thin, with a height running along the 97th centile (and head circumference on the 90th). In view of his educational problems, notably with writing and reading, and his tall stature (though this was in fact similar to that of his two brothers), chromosome analysis was undertaken, revealing a karyotype of 47,XXY. On examination at the age of 10 he was a pleasant, quiet, cooperative boy, noted to have proportionately long legs, but normal prepubertal genitalia, though the testes, which were both lying in the scrotum, were very small. His bone age was advanced by about a year, but by the age of $11\frac{3}{4}$ there was no evidence of imminent puberty and he was started on low dose testosterone therapy. He has not developed gynaecomastia.

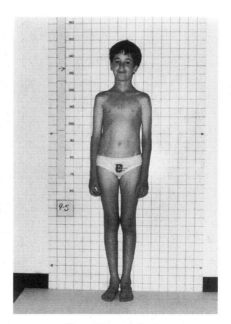

Case 32 at 9·5 years

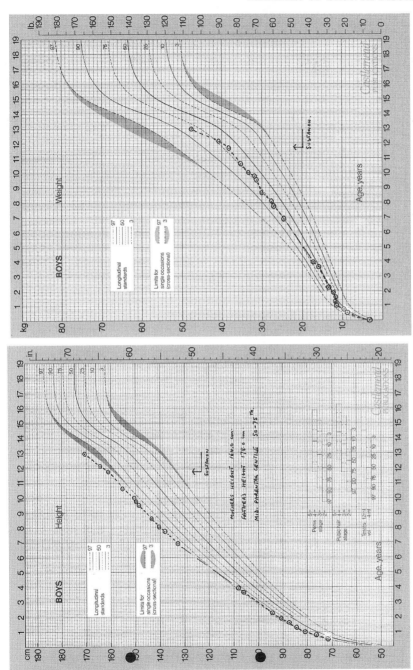

Case 32 (height and weight charts)

175

33 In contrast to the patient above, the diagnosis of Klinefelter's syndrome was made on chromosomal analysis shortly after the birth of this boy because he was noted to have micropenis. He was a large baby (4200 g at term) and has grown rapidly with a height at the age of $8\frac{1}{2}$ years above the 97th centile, and weight not much dissimilar. At the age of $3\frac{3}{4}$ he was given testosterone treatment for two months, which resulted in good growth of the penis; this was prior to surgery undertaken to redistribute the skin following circumcision.

His development throughout has been entirely normal, with appropriate milestones and performance well up to average in a normal school. Measurements show him to have long legs and his testes remain very small. His bone age is appropriate for his chronological age.

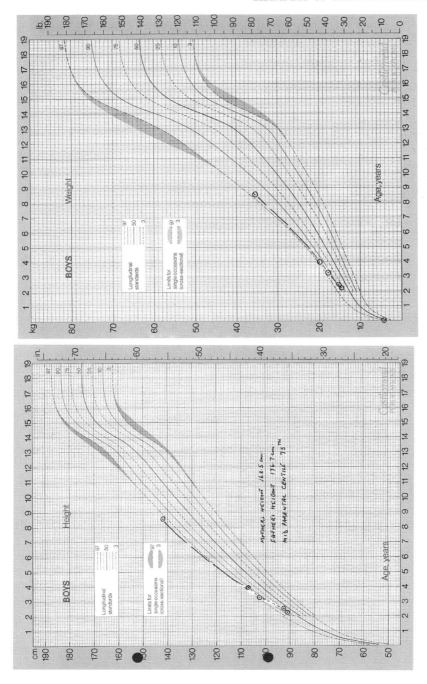

Case 33 (height and weight charts)

177

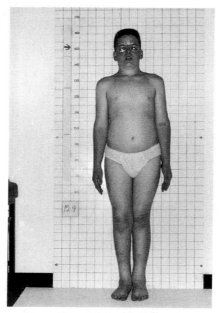

Case 34 at 12·9 years

XYY CHROMOSOME ANOMALY

34 This young man had presented at the age of $7\frac{1}{2}$ years with grand mal seizures and severe behavioural disturbance. This was manifest as immaturity, with disobedience, attention seeking, temper tantrums, and aggression towards other children, and became worse on anticonvulsant treatment. He had been demanding from birth, and slow both developmentally and intellectually. He was of a normal size at birth, weighing 3320 g at term, and was not particularly tall in early childhood, though relatively obese. He reached puberty at an earlier than average age, with marked acceleration in his growth, and he developed severely inappropriate sexual behaviour directed against both sexes and of any age. These features improved dramatically with treatment with cyproterone, which slowed down the progress of puberty.

This case illustrates the minority of XYY individuals in which characteristic abnormalities of growth and behaviour do seem to be linked with the chromosomal abnormality.

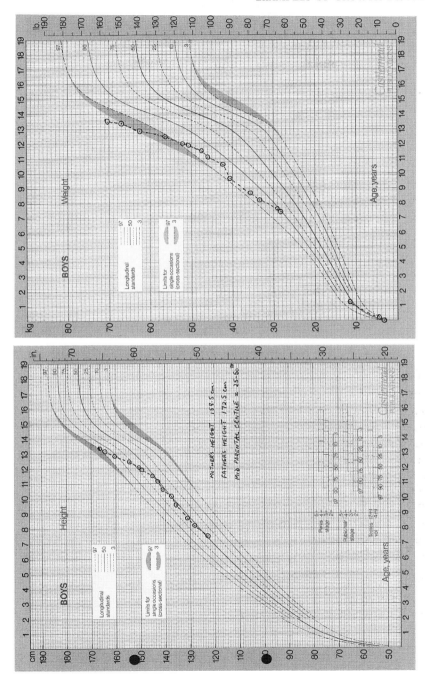

Case 34 (height and weight charts)

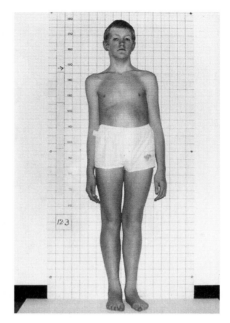

Case 35 at 12·3 years

SOTOS SYNDROME

35 This boy was large at birth, weighing 4500 g at term, following a pregnancy in which his mother was severely hypertensive in the last trimester. He was floppy and lethargic in the neonatal period, with episodes of hypoglycaemia, and required tube feeding. He had a large head with a circumference greater than the 97th centile, which it has continued to be.

His developmental milestones were delayed, with poor coordination, and subsequent assessment identified the need for special education.

He was referred at the age of 12 because of his extreme tallness. In addition to his low intelligence and lack of coordination, he was noted to be very long limbed with arachnodactyly and hyperextensible joints. He had a high forehead, prominent chin, and high arched palate. He had a severe lower thoracic scoliosis, convex to the right with accentuated lumbar lordosis. Bone age was markedly advanced, being 15·3 years at an age of 12·3, and the metacarpal index was very high (11) (as reported

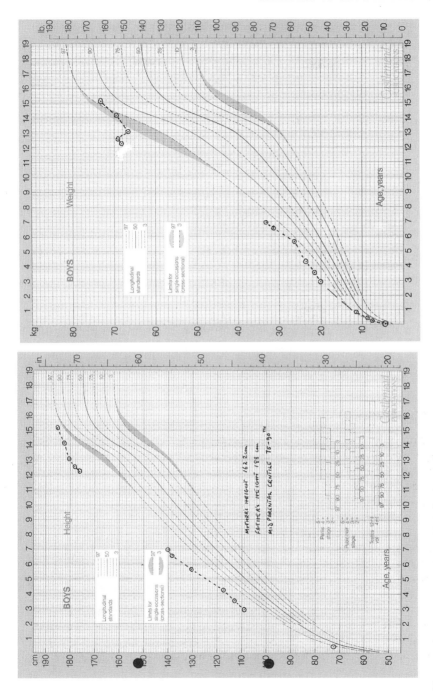

Chart 35 (height and weight charts)

181

in Sotos syndrome). There were no abnormalities in the eyes or heart. Endocrine investigations were normal.

He was at an early stage of puberty, which has subsequently progressed fast, and at the age of 15 he is nearly fully grown with almost adult bone age.

References

1 *Boys and girls growth standards*. London: Child Growth Foundation, 1994.
2 *Boys and girls: birth–19 years. Height and weight. Tanner–Whitehouse growth and development records*. Welwyn Garden City, UK: Castlemead Publications, 1975.
   Tanner JM, Whitehouse RH. Clinical longitudinal standards for height, weight, height velocity, weight velocity and stages of puberty. *Arch Dis Child* 1976; **51**: 170–9.
3 Gairdner D., Pearson J. A growth chart for premature and other infants. *Arch Dis Child* 1971; **46**: 783–7.
4 Tanner JM. Physical growth and development. In: Forfar JO, Arneil GC (eds) *Textbook of paediatrics*, 3rd edn. Edinburgh: Churchill Livingstone, 1984, pp 278–330.
5 Buckler JMH. *A longitudinal study of adolescent growth*. London: Springer-Verlag, 1990.
6 Hall DMB (ed) *Health for all children*, 2nd edn. Oxford: Oxford Medical Publications, 1991.
7 Cameron N. The methods of auxological anthropometry. In: Falkner F, Tanner JM (eds) *Human growth. A comprehensive treatise*, vol 3, 2nd edn. New York: Plenum Press, 1986, pp 3–46.
8 Tanner JM. *Growth at adolescence*, 2nd edn. Oxford: Blackwell Scientific, 1962.
9 Buckler JMH. *A reference manual of growth and development*. Oxford: Blackwell Scientific, 1979.
10 Buckler JMH, Green M. Birth weight and head circumference standards for English twins. *Arch Dis Child* (In press).
11 Buckler JMH, Buckler J. Growth characteristics in twins and higher order multiple births. *Acta Genet Med Gemellol (Roma)* 1987; **36**: 197–208.
12 Wilson RS. Growth standards for twins from birth to four years. *Ann Hum Biol* 1974; **1**: 175–88.
13 Pyle SI, Waterhouse AM, Greulich WW. *A radiographic standard of reference for the growing hand and wrist*. Chicago: Press of Case Western Reserve University (Yearbook Medical Publishers), 1971.
14 Tanner JM, Whitehouse RH, Cameron N, Marshall WA, Healy MJR, Goldstein H. *Assessment of skeletal maturity and prediction of adult height*, 2nd edn. London: Academic Press, 1983.
15 Skuse D. Psychological consequence of being small. *J Child Psychol* 1987; **28**: 641–50.

General

1 Brook CGD. *Clinical paediatric endocrinology*, 2nd edn. Oxford: Blackwell Scientific, 1989.
2 Brook CGD. *A guide to the practice of paediatric endocrinology*. Cambridge: Cambridge University Press, 1993.
3 Marshall WA, Tanner JM. Puberty. In: Falkner F, Tanner JM (eds) *Human growth. A comprehensive treatise*, vol 3, 2nd edn. New York: Plenum Press, pp 171–209.
4 Tanner JM. Physical growth and development. In: Forfar JO, Arneil GC (eds) *Textbook of paediatrics*, 3rd edn. Edinburgh: Churchill Livingstone, 1984, pp 278–330.

Appendix 1: Suppliers

Measuring equipment

Many instruments are available for measurement of weight, length, and height with a wide range in price, reliability, ease of use, and mobility. Advice and information including price lists can be obtained from:

(1) The Child Growth Foundation,
     2 Mayfield Avenue,
     Chiswick,
     London W4 IPW

(2) Castlemead Publications,
     12 Little Mundells,
     Welwyn Garden City,
     Hertfordshire AL7 IEW

More expensive precision apparatus for measuring height, length and skinfolds are available from:

Holtain Ltd,
Crosswell,
Crymmych,
Pembrokeshire

and for weight:

Halifax Scale Company,
Brighouse Road,
Hipperholme,
Halifax HX3 8EF

Wall height screening charts, many of the weighing scales, and the Prader orchidometer are obtainable from the Child Growth Foundation at the address given above.

Appendix 2: Growth charts

The following are obtainable from Castlemead Publications (address given in Appendix 1):

British Standards (Tanner–Whitehouse)
  Height and Weight
  Height and Weight Velocity
  Head Circumference
  Sitting Height and Leg Length
  Triceps and Subscapular Skinfolds

Gairdner–Pearson Standards
  Growth Records for Premature and Other Infants: Length, Weight and Head Circumference

North American Standards (Tanner–Davies)
  Height and Height Velocity

Irish Standards (Hoey–Tanner–Cox)
  Height and Weight and Height Velocity

Down's Syndrome Centiles
Turner's Syndrome Centiles

Current UK Cross Sectional Standards
  Weight, Length/Height (0–18 years) and Head Circumference (in infancy) are obtainable from the Child Growth Foundation (address given in Appendix 1).

Appendix 3: Normal Values

These may vary to a minor degree between laboratories

Basic biochemistry (Serum or plasma)

Sodium	135–145 mmol/l
Potassium	3·6–5·0 mmol/l
Chloride	98–107 mmol/l
Bicarbonate	21–28 mmol/l
Urea	2·5–7·1 mmol/l
Creatinine	50–120 μmol/l

Calcium homeostasis (Plasma)

Calcium	2·25–2·60 mmol/l
Phosphate	0·80–1·30 mmol/l — adults
	0·60–1·80 mmol/l — children
Alkaline phosphatase	100–300 IU/l — adults
	values higher in children and linked to growth rate
Parathyroid hormone	<1·0 ng/ml
25-hydroxycholecalciferol	8–40 ng/ml

Glucose homeostasis (Plasma)

Fasting glucose	3·5–6·0 mmol/l
Glycosylated haemoglobin (HbA$_1$C)	5·7–8·0%
Insulin	<10 mU/l (when glucose is normal or low)

Hypothalamo-pituitary axis (Plasma)

Growth hormone	Basal low < 10 mU/l
	Peak post stimulation — exercise
	> 15 mU/l other stimuli > 20 mU/l
Thyroid stimulating	Basal 0·2–6·0 mU/l
hormone (TSH)	Peak following thyrotropin releasing
	hormone (TRH), usually about 12 at 20
	minutes
Prolactin	<500 mU/l unstimulated
Adrenocorticotropic	Basal 0900 hrs < 80 ng/l
hormone (ACTH)	Midnight < 10 ng/l
Antidiuretic hormone	Basal 1–5 pmol/l
(ADH)	
Plasma osmolality	275–295 mosm/kg water (< 295 on fluid
	deprivation)
Urine osmolality	> 750 mosm/kg water on fluid deprivation
Luteinising hormone	Basal prepubertal low < 1·5 IU/l
(LH)	Basal pubertal rises through puberty
	progressively to about 8 IU/l
	Post luteinising releasing hormone (LRH)
	—rises at all ages, greater in puberty
	eg, prepubertal to about 4 IU/l
	pubertal to about 20 IU/l
	Adult male <10 IU/l
	female — depends on phase of menstrual
	cycle
Follicle stimulating	Basal prepubertal low <2·0 IU/l
hormone (FSH)	Basal pubertal rises to about 2·5 IU/l
	Post luteinising releasing hormone (LRH)
	rises at all ages to about 5 IU/l
	Adult male < 8 IU/l
	female < 8 IU/l

Thyroid (Plasma)

Total T4	60–150 nmol/l
Total T3	1·2–3·1 nmol/l
Free T4	10–30 pmol/l
Free T3	3–9 pmol/l
Thyroid stimulating hormone (TSH)	see above

Adrenal cortex (Plasma)

Cortisol

Basal 0900 hrs		100–600 nmol/l
midnight		< 300 nmol/l (about 50% morning values)
17 α-hydroxyprogesterone	in prepuberty	< 15 nmol/l
	adults	< 10 nmol/l
11-deoxycortisol		< 60 nmol/l
Androstenedione	children	< 3·5 nmol/l
	adult female	3·0–12·0 nmol/l
	adult male	2·0–10·0 nmol/l
Dehydroepiandrosterone sulphate	prepubertal	< 1 μmol/l
	adult female	3·0–11·0 μmol/l
	adult male	4·0–13·0 μmol/l
Plasma renin activity	infants	< 5 pmol/ml/hour — falling to adult range by age 8 years
	children	recumbent
	> 8 yrs and adults	1·1–2·7 pmol/ml/hour ambulant 2.8–4·5 pmol/ml/hour

Adrenal cortex (Urine)

17 oxosteroids	infants	< 3 μmol/day
	children	<12 μmol/day
	adult female	10–70 μmol/day
	male	20–100 μmol/day
Pregnanetriol	infant	<0·3 μmol/day
	children	< 3 μmol/day
	adults	1·5–6·0 μmol/day
Urinary free cortisol		< 350 nmol/day
11-oxygenation index		< 0·7 (seldom used now)

Gonads (Plasma)

Luteinising hormone (LH) and follicle stimulating hormone (FSH)	see above	
Testosterone	prepubertal	< 0·9 nmol/l
	adult female	0·5–2·5 nmol/l
	adult male	8–27 nmol/l

Post human chorionic gonadotrophin (HCG) stimulation (at 48 hours) reaches adult levels at any age

Oestradiol	prepubertal	< 60 pmol/l
	adult male	< 150 pmol/l
	adult female	200–2000 pmol/l (depending on phase of menstrual cycle)
Progesterone	prepubertal	< 1·3 nmol/l
	adult male	< 1·3 nmol/l
	adult female	< 5 nmol/l — follicular phase of cycle
		6–60 nmol/l — luteal phase of cycle

Index